10/5/23

THE
VEGAN
STARTER
KIT

ALSO BY **NEAL D. BARNARD, MD, FACC**

The Power of Your Plate

A Physician's Slimming Guide

Food for Life

Eat Right, Live Longer

Foods That Fight Pain

Turn Off the Fat Genes

Breaking the Food Seduction

Nutrition Guide for Clinicians

The Cancer Survivor's Guide

Dr. Neal Barnard's Program for Reversing Diabetes

21-Day Weight Loss Kickstart

Power Foods for the Brain

The Cheese Trap

THE VEGAN STARTER KIT

EVERYTHING YOU NEED TO KNOW ABOUT PLANT-BASED EATING

NEAL D. BARNARD, MD, FACC

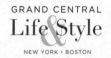

GRAND CENTRAL
Life & Style
NEW YORK · BOSTON

Copyright © 2018 by Neal D. Barnard, MD, FACC
Cover design by Amy Sly
Cover copyright © 2018 by Hachette Book Group, Inc.

Grand Central Life & Style
Hachette Book Group
1290 Avenue of the Americas, New York, NY 10104
grandcentrallifeandstyle.com
twitter.com/grandcentralpub

First Edition: December 2018

Grand Central Life & Style is an imprint of Grand Central Publishing. The Grand Central Life & Style name and logo are trademarks of Hachette Book Group, Inc.

The publisher is not responsible for websites (or their content) that are not owned by the publisher.

The Hachette Speakers Bureau provides a wide range of authors for speaking events. To find out more, go to www.hachettespeakersbureau.com or call (866) 376-6591.

Print book interior design by Fearn Cutler de Vicq

Library of Congress Cataloging-in-Publication Data

Names: Barnard, Neal D.
Title: The vegan starter kit / Neal D. Barnard, MD, FACC.
Description: First edition. | New York, NY: Grand Central Life & Style, [2018] | Includes bibliographical references and index.
Identifiers: LCCN 2018022906| ISBN 9781538747407 (trade pbk.) | ISBN 9781549171222 (audio download) | ISBN 9781538747414 (ebook)
Subjects: LCSH: Vegetarianism. | Nutrition. | Health. | Vegan cooking. | LCGFT: Cookbooks.
Classification: LCC RM236 .B359 2018 | DDC 641.5/636—dc23
LC record available at https://lccn.loc.gov/2018022906

Printed in the United States of America

LSC-C

10 9 8 7 6 5 4 3 2 1

꒰ • ꒱

Contents

A Note to the Reader

THIS BOOK WILL INTRODUCE YOU TO THE POWER OF VEGAN FOODS. It's easy to put that power to work, and the payoff is huge, as you will soon see! Even so, let me mention two important points:

☞ **If you have a health condition or use medications, see your health care provider.** Often, people need less medication when they improve their diets. This is common for people who have diabetes or high blood pressure, for example. Sometimes, they can discontinue their drugs altogether. But do not change your medications on your own. Work with your health care provider to reduce or discontinue your medicines if and when the time is right.

☞ **Get complete nutrition.** Plant-based foods are the most nutritious foods there are. Even so, you will want to ensure that you get complete nutrition. To do that, include a variety of vegetables, fruits, whole grains, and legumes in your routine, and I would suggest a special focus on green leafy vegetables. And be sure to have a reliable source of vitamin B_{12} daily, such as a simple B_{12} supplement. Vitamin B_{12} is essential for healthy nerves and healthy blood. You will find more details in Chapter 5.

THE
VEGAN
STARTER
KIT

MILLIONS OF PEOPLE ARE LOOKING AT VEGAN CHOICES. Some aim to lose weight, improve their health, or boost their athletic ability. Others are motivated by compassion for animals or concern for the environment. Many are intrigued by the cool new vegan products at supermarkets, health food stores, restaurants, and fast-food spots.

Whether you want to just test out vegan eating for a week or two or plan to stick with it permanently, you no doubt have questions: How do I plan a meal? Am I getting complete nutrition? How do I cook when I'm pressed for time (without spending a fortune at the health food store)? How do I find good meals on the road? Do I need supplements?

This book will answer those questions and many more and will show you how to begin. It was inspired by a magazine-style booklet called the *Vegetarian Starter Kit*, first published by the Physicians Committee for Responsible Medicine in the 1990s. That guide proved extraordinarily popular. Stacks of them quickly vanished from doctors' waiting rooms, convention booths, and health fairs, scooped up by people who were attracted by plant-based eating and were delighted to find a reliable guide to get them started. The format was quickly copied by many other organizations. This book retains the simplicity of the magazine-style booklet but adds lots of practical details to make going vegan easy and fun. It is called a "kit" because it has everything you need to get started, including thorough answers to common questions, details on ensuring complete nutrition during childhood, pregnancy, and other stages of life, and quick-reference charts, as well as a complete starter set of easy and delicious recipes and tips for modifying recipes of your own, among many other features.

>> In case you are wondering about terminology, let me help you. A *vegan* diet simply means there are no animal products on the menu—no meat, dairy, or eggs. "Vegetarian" means meatless, so a vegetarian meal might be vegan or might not, depending on whether it includes cheese or other dairy products. Some people use the term "plant-based," which nowadays is synonymous with "vegan." Some say "whole-foods plant-based," meaning they not only are skipping animal products but are generally preferring whole grains and other intact foods over processed foods, such as sugar, flour, and the like. <<

Uh-oh, you may be thinking. "Do I have to learn to cook?" The answer is no. A vegan diet will improve your health, but it won't change your personality. If you are too impatient to cook now, that's not likely to change. So we'll include plenty of tips for keeping things simple. That said, there are advantages to being able to decide what goes into the foods you're eating, so do have a look at the recipes.

This guide has everything you need to jump into a healthful vegan diet (and we'll use "plant-based" as a synonym for it). You will learn how to maximize the benefits for specific health conditions and how to make it work on the job and when you travel. We'll also tackle some common bumps in the road and common myths.

As you will see, a vegan diet is the easiest and healthiest way to lose weight and keep it off for good. And for people with high cholesterol, high blood pressure, or diabetes, it is a powerful way to turn these conditions around. It can help you reverse heart disease, reduce your cancer risk, and cut your risk of Alzheimer's disease.

Soon you'll find that going vegan is easy and is very powerful for your health. It is also an adventure. Rather than being the extreme end of a diet exploration, going vegan will feel like a healthy new beginning. Once you've gotten the animal products off your plate, you'll want to explore many more things. There are wonderful cuisines from around the world, endless new foods to try, innovative websites, and lots of books, movies, and recipes to share. Along with them come more and more health benefits.

Please share the information you find here with anyone and everyone you know. You'll love it, and they will, too!

CHAPTER 1

The Best Decision
I Ever Made

THERE ARE ENORMOUS HEALTH ADVANTAGES TO GOING VEGAN. For starters, it makes it easy to lose weight without cutting calories or going hungry. Whether you would like to lose twenty pounds or two hundred, this is the easiest way to drop that weight and to keep it off for good. Plant-based eating brings many other welcome changes, too!

Heart disease reverses. In 1990, Dean Ornish, MD, of the Preventive Medicine Research Institute and the University of California, San Francisco, showed that a vegetarian diet, along with other lifestyle changes, *reversed* heart disease in 82 percent of research subjects in one year, without medications or surgery.

Cholesterol levels improve. A vegan diet is the most powerful eating plan for cutting cholesterol. Unlike a Mediterranean diet, a low-carbohydrate diet, or any other diet approach, a vegan diet eliminates *all* the cholesterol and animal fat from foods, and it includes specific cholesterol-lowering nutrients. More on this in Chapter 4.

High blood pressure improves. A detailed review published by the American Medical Association showed that plant-based eating effectively reduces blood pressure, both because it avoids the blood-pressure-raising effect of animal products and because it takes advantage of special blood-pressure-lowering nutrients found in plants.

Diabetes gets better and sometimes goes away altogether. In 2003, the National Institutes of Health funded our research team at the Physicians Committee for Responsible Medicine to do a head-to-head test of a low-fat vegan diet versus a conventional "diabetes diet" that relied on cutting calories and limiting carbohydrates for people with type 2 diabetes. Every week, the research participants came to our office to learn about healthful foods, to sit in on cooking demonstrations, and to discuss their successes and challenges. And as the weeks went by, remarkable things happened. Weight loss began immediately and effortlessly. Without counting calories or limiting portions, our participants started to trim away pounds. Blood sugars that had been stuck in the danger zone began to fall, as did cholesterol levels and blood pressure. And many participants were able to reduce their medicines or stop them completely. Compared with a conventional "diabetes diet," the vegan diet turned out to be three times more powerful at controlling blood sugar and even improved long-standing problems, such as painful diabetic nerve symptoms.

Painful conditions, such as arthritis, migraines, and menstrual cramps, often diminish or simply go away. The menu adjustment you are making removes animal-derived products that can inflame joints and trigger migraines, and also brings hormones into a healthier balance.

Cancer risk falls, and people previously diagnosed with cancer are better able to keep their cancer at bay. This appears to be especially true of digestive cancers, such as colorectal cancer, and hormonal cancers, such as breast and prostate cancer. Overall, people following plant-based diets cut their cancer risk as much as 40 percent.

Alzheimer's disease is less likely to strike, according to the best evidence we have. The disease is much more common among people eating more *saturated* fat—that is, the "bad" fat found in dairy products and meat—while people following plant-based diets appear to be better able to preserve their memory and cognitive abilities as the years go by.

As these conditions improve, you may find that you need less medication or none at all. Less medicine means fewer side effects and less expense. And it means you are getting at the *cause* of these problems, not just treating them with a pharmaceutical Band-Aid.

For people trying to knock off some weight, or who have been in and out of doctors' offices and are taking a seemingly endless list of medicines, or who just want to start down a better path, a menu change is welcome relief. It gives you power you didn't know you could have.

Everyone's Talking About It

When Bill Clinton, Ellen DeGeneres, and a steady stream of other celebrities began to embrace vegan or nearly vegan diets, it was clear that plant-based eating had reached prime time. The US government officially recognized the health value of vegan diets in the 2015 *Dietary Guidelines for Americans,* as did the American Medical Association, the Academy of Nutrition and Dietetics, and countless health experts. The United Nations weighed in on the power of plant-based eating for the environment. People concerned about animals, of course, have been going vegan for many years.

The latest wave is in the world of sports. Elite runners, including Carl Lewis, Scott Jurek, Brendan Brazier, Rich Roll, and Fiona

Oakes, started the trend, using vegan diets to boost blood flow and oxygenation of their muscles for better endurance and to take advantage of a vegan diet's anti-inflammatory effect to speed their post-workout recovery. When tennis star Venus Williams was diagnosed with Sjögren's syndrome, an autoimmune condition, a vegan diet helped her defeat the condition and get back into winning form. Her sister Serena followed her dietary lead. Basketball and football players are using the power of plants to replace flab with muscle, boost their performance, and extend their careers. In 2017, racing champion Lewis Hamilton went vegan before winning his fourth Formula One World Drivers' Championship, saying he felt "the best I have ever felt in my life, in my thirty-two years." Olympic snowboarding medalist Hannah Teter said that a plant-based diet brought her performance to "a whole other level." Tia Blanco won the Open Women's World Surfing Championship two years in a row after ditching meat and dairy.

And It Gets Better

A vegan diet is great, not just for health, but also for animals. Currently, Americans eat about a million animals *every hour*, and their lives on the way to slaughter are enough to make anyone wince. A vegan diet is a big vote for compassion.

It is also a vote for the environment. There are currently nearly 100 million cattle in the United States alone, and each one is as big as a sofa. They are continually belching methane—a potent greenhouse gas—into the atmosphere. And fattening them up—along with pigs and chickens—requires an enormous amount of feed grain, which means huge quantities of water, fertilizer, and pesticides that despoil our rivers and streams. A plant-based diet means much less impact on the environment.

It is also great for your loved ones. One of the kindest things you can do is to help them improve their eating habits; you may even save their lives. If you have children, a vegan diet will protect their health, teach them important values, and preserve the Earth they will one day inherit. And when you follow a healthful diet yourself, you are helping to ensure that you will be there for them when they need you.

Okay, but how about taste? You'll soon discover that your new array of healthful foods turns out to be the best you've ever had. When I was growing up in Fargo, North Dakota, our eating habits were nothing to brag about. Our daily fare was roast beef, potatoes, and an obligatory vegetable. Sometimes a chicken leg might end up on the plate, and a salad might raise its head now and again. But I never heard anyone say they just adored Fargo-style cuisine. "Wow, let's launch a restaurant of all the Fargo favorites!" It was food; that was all.

After moving to Washington, DC, I had the chance to discover the culinary treasures of other lands, many of them drawing their ingredients from healthful plant-based staples. Italian restaurants featured piping-hot bowls of minestrone or lentil soup, followed by angel hair pasta topped with arrabbiata sauce with garlic-roasted asparagus or sautéed spinach on the side. Mexican restaurants served spicy bean burritos, veggie fajitas, and fresh guacamole. Japanese restaurants offered miso soup, exotic salads, and vegan sushi rolls made of cucumber and avocado. Szechuan and Hunan restaurants cooked up every possible dish made from vegetables, tofu, and rice, all delicately spiced. Other restaurants were inspired by the traditions of France, Spain, India, Greece, Cuba, Lebanon, Vietnam,

Thailand, Ethiopia, and many other lands. All of them are able to turn simple vegetables, fruits, beans, and grains into delicacies. In comparison to these delights, my North Dakota beef and potatoes seemed a bit pedestrian.

> ➤ In addition to taste, I discovered one more advantage of healthful plant-based eating. The cleanup is amazingly quick. You're not scrubbing a roast pan coated with what seems like baked-on asphalt or digging out a grease-clogged drain. That may sound trivial. But if it takes a lot of elbow grease to clean out a pan, imagine what that food is doing inside your body. When you follow a vegan diet, there is much less need for surgeons to clean out your arteries or intestinal tract! ➤

So, going vegan really is the best decision you could ever make. For your heart, your waistline, your overall health, the animals, the Earth, and your loved ones. It is just what the doctor ordered. So jump in and see what the power of healthy eating can do for you.

CHAPTER 2

It's Really That Easy!

OING VEGAN IS EASY. IT'S EASIER THAN GOING LOW-CARB or gluten-free. And it's much easier than quitting smoking or breaking other habits. Because you can eat as much as you want. You are never counting calories or carb grams. Yes, a vegan diet does mean skipping animal products—meat, dairy products, and eggs— but there are plenty of great things to take their place.

There are really only two "rules":

1. Build your meals from plant-based foods, especially vegetables, fruits, whole grains, and legumes (beans, peas, and lentils).
2. Ensure complete nutrition with a supplement of vitamin B_{12}.

That's it. Those are the "rules." Let's take a closer look.

The first "rule" guides you to replace animal products with the four healthful food groups that are nutrition powerhouses: vegetables, fruits, whole grains, and legumes. These are your palette. In the same way that a master painter combines simple colors to create a masterpiece, our simple four food groups combine to make delicious meals that bring you the best possible health. Let's look at each food group.

Vegetables. Everyone knows that vegetables are loaded with vitamins and minerals. But that's just for starters. They are also surprisingly high in protein. Take broccoli. It's about one-third protein, as a percentage of its calories. Spinach is about 50 percent protein. The amount varies from one vegetable to another, but you get the idea. Bison, horses, elephants, giraffes, and many other animals build their massive musculature entirely from plants.

Instead of making vegetables a mere side dish, put them front and center. And why not have two at a meal, say, a green vegetable and an orange vegetable, like broccoli and sweet potatoes, or spinach and carrots?

The Power Plate

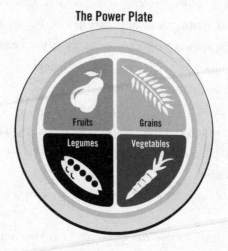

Fruits. Fruits are loaded with vitamins, of course. But they are also rich in fiber to tame your appetite, and their natural sugars are surprisingly easy on your blood sugar.

Whole grains. Rice, oats, wheat, corn, quinoa, and the full range of other grains bring you healthful complex carbohydrates for energy and a significant amount of protein. And each grain has a natural fiber coating. Although food manufacturers often remove it to turn brown rice into white rice and whole-grain bread into white bread, you are better off leaving the fiber in place. Not only are grains more flavorful in their original package but fiber is a cancer fighter and keeps your digestion running smoothly.

Legumes. Beans, peas, and lentils bring you protein, iron, calcium, fiber, and healthful complex carbohydrates for energy.

On your plate, vegetables, fruits, legumes, and grains turn into a breakfast of blueberry pancakes with maple syrup, oatmeal with cinnamon and raisins, a breakfast scramble, or veggie sausage. For lunch they transform into split pea soup with a hummus sandwich, hearty chili, or a veggie stir-fry. For dinner these simple food groups make a savory stew, shepherd's pie, veggie sushi, vegetable pizza, a tasty curry, or thousands of other delicious possibilities.

⋙ **You may also wish to add some nuts, seeds, or olives. They are low in "bad" fats and cholesterol-free. But I would suggest that you go easy. Even though the fat they hold is much more healthful than animal fats, they are still calorie-dense. More on this in Chapter 4.** ⋘

The second "rule" is to ensure complete nutrition with a supplement of vitamin B_{12}. We'll cover this in more detail in Chapter 5. For now, it's important to know that you need B_{12} for healthy nerves and healthy blood, and that it is not made by either animals or plants. It is made by bacteria. So the bacteria in a cow's gut make some B_{12} that ends up in meat and milk. On a vegan diet you'll need to get B_{12} either as a supplement (available in all drugstores and natural food stores) or from fortified foods (e.g., B_{12}-fortified soy milk).

So those are the "rules." In the next chapter we'll look at how to get started and we'll see what delicious masterpieces we can create.

CHAPTER 3

How to Start

OKAY, IT'S TIME TO BEGIN! IN OUR RESEARCH STUDIES, WE break the diet change into two easy steps, and I have never seen anyone unable to do this:

Step 1: Take a week to check out the possibilities. Our goal is to identify vegan foods that you really like (many of which are already familiar, as you'll see) and to check out the great new ways to substitute meats and cheeses. A surprising array of delicious foods awaits you, and now is the time to pick out your favorites.

On a sheet of paper, make headings for breakfast, lunch, dinner, and snacks. Your job for the next seven days is to fill in your paper with foods that are free of animal products that you would like to bring into your routine. For now, don't eliminate anything from your diet. Just think about vegan foods that you already enjoy or would like to try. Jot them down, and try them this week. If you haven't had oatmeal since you were a kid and have been meaning to try it again, now's the time. Top it with cinnamon and raisins or sliced strawberries, or whatever will make it tasty. If you like it, keep it on your list. If not, cross it off and try a different breakfast item. How about trying almond milk with your morning cereal or coffee? If you eat sausage in the morning but have never tasted veggie sausage, how about picking some up at the store to see what you think? Write these ideas down. If you like them, keep them. If not, try a different brand or cross them off your list.

Consider adding a soup to your lunch routine: minestrone, butternut squash, lentil, tomato, vegetarian vegetable, or other flavor. For convenience, canned varieties are at every natural food store and many regular grocery stores. Check the labels, and skip any that are made with milk or other animal products. Or how about a salad of baby spinach, mixed greens, chopped tomatoes, olives, and shredded carrots, topped with balsamic vinaigrette? Premade salads are fine. Add a hummus sandwich, a veggie stir-fry, a veggie hot dog, or whatever calls to you.

> ➤ **Make your green vegetables extra delicious with a spritz of Bragg Liquid Aminos, seasoned rice vinegar, or lemon juice.** ◄

Think about the foods you already like that happen to be vegan, and put them on your list.

For inspiration, have a look at the recipes in this book. And try new products at the grocery store and new restaurant options—Italian, Mexican, Chinese, Japanese, Ethiopian, Indian, or whatever you like. The goal is to come up with vegan meal ideas that you'll want to stick with. As you will see, there are lots of great choices.

⚓ *Breakfast*

_____

_____

_____

_____

⚓ *Lunch*

_____

_____

_____

_____

⚓ *Dinner*

_____

_____

_____

_____

⚓ *Snacks*

_____

_____

_____

_____

HEALTHY

Breakfast Ideas

Bircher Muesli (page 109)

Carrot Cake Muffins (page 110)

Easy Tofu Scramble (page 111)

Cinnamon raisin oatmeal

Blueberry pancakes

French toast

Corn flakes with almond milk and banana slices

Veggie sausage, veggie bacon

Whole-grain bagel with jam

Breakfast burrito
filled with refried beans, lettuce, and tomato

Fresh cantaloupe melon, bananas,
and blueberries

HEALTHY

Lunches and Dinners

Soups: lentil, butternut squash, Minestrone (page 121),
tomato, split pea, vegetable

Pasta e Fagioli (page 123)

Quick Black Bean Chili (page 125)

Sandwich of Super-Quick Hummus (page 127) with lettuce and tomato

Lasagna (page 130)

Easy Stuffed Peppers (page 130)

Pasta Bowl with Beans and Greens (page 132)

Spaghetti Alfredo (page 133)

Pizza with mushrooms, onions, spinach, sundried tomatoes

Bean burrito

Baked beans with veggie-dog chunks

Submarine sandwich with lettuce, tomato, cucumber,
olives, and sautéed mushrooms on a toasted bun

Veggie or portobello mushroom burgers, veggie hot dogs

Three-bean salad

Mandarin vegetable stir-fry

Step 2: After testing out foods for a week, you're getting a sense of which ones you like. Now, for the next three weeks, make your meals all vegan all the time, using the foods that you have already picked out. During this time, do not have any animal products at all. It's only three weeks; focusing on just choosing the foods that you like one meal at a time will make it feel easy. And let me share a few tips to make your twenty-one-day "test drive" extra easy:

1. Feel free to use "transition foods." There are excellent substitutes for burgers, hot dogs, sausage, and ground beef for use in chili or spaghetti sauce, among others, and there are many substitutes for milk and other dairy products.

2. Be strict. Just as smokers find it easier to quit completely than to tease themselves with an occasional cigarette, people getting away from meat and dairy products find it easier to skip these products entirely. Even the occasional bit of fried chicken or cheese will lure your taste buds back to unhealthful foods. So keep your "test drive" 100 percent vegan.

3. Focus on the short term. Don't worry about what you will do a year from now. Just focus on a three-week experiment.

Look for support from loved ones. Any change of routine is easier with a little moral support. Ask your friends and family to join you in a short-term diet experiment. Or if they choose not to, you can ask them to support you in what you are doing and not to tease you or tempt you with unhealthful foods. Eventually, they'll see the value of what you are doing and may well decide to join you.

By the end of twenty-one days, you will notice two things: First, you are healthier. You're losing unwanted pounds, your energy is better, and your digestion is improving. If you have diabetes, you may notice that your blood sugar is getting better day by day. The same is true for cholesterol and blood pressure. Second, you'll find that your tastes are changing. You're losing your desire for unhealthful foods and are really coming to love your new foods.

After your three-week "test drive," you are free to do whatever you want. But chances are you'll want to stick with it. Your health benefits will continue to grow, and your exploration of new foods will be more and more rewarding. Soon it will all be second nature. And you are now taking real health power into your hands.

Quick Substitutes

You really don't need a literal replacement for meat. Pasta dishes, cheese-free pizza, curries, and stir-fries all go great without even thinking about meat. That goes for dairy products and eggs, too. You can just skip them. But if you want something to replace meat, dairy products, and eggs, here are some ideas:

Replacing Meat

Beans work great in chili, tacos, spaghetti sauces, and curries. Like meat, they are protein-rich, but they are free of animal fat and cholesterol.

Tempeh, made from fermented soybeans and sold in natural food stores and Asian markets, works as a substitute for breakfast meats (see the Breakfast Grillers recipe, page 112) or in stir-fries.

Veggie burgers or **veggie dogs** are available at most grocery stores. They are quick, convenient, and popular with kids. Portobello mushrooms also make great substitutes for burgers.

Vegan sausage is nearly indistinguishable from the porcine variety and is *much* better for you. Veggie bacon is a more liberal interpretation of the original, but try a few brands and see what you think.

Replacing Dairy Products

Nondairy products are now widely available. They come in a huge variety of flavors, so try a few to see which ones you like.

Milk has met its match with soy milk, rice milk, almond milk, oat milk, hemp milk, and many other varieties. Some are fortified with calcium and vitamin B_{12}.

Nondairy yogurts are made from almonds, cashews, soybeans, and other ingredients.

Frozen desserts started with sorbet and have exploded into a huge range of ice cream substitutes, including several from major ice cream brands.

Vegan cheeses and **sour cream** are available at natural food stores. They are fatty and should be thought of as occasional treats.

Nutritional yeast lends a cheesy flavor to pizza, spaghetti sauce, vegetables, and casseroles.

Avocado chunks replace feta when you're topping a salad.

Replacing Eggs

A single egg has as much cholesterol as an 8-ounce steak, along with plenty of fat and animal protein. Luckily, replacing eggs is easy.

Instead of scrambled eggs, try scrambled tofu (see the Easy Tofu Scramble recipe, page 111). Tofu has a texture almost identical to egg white, and scrambled tofu quickly becomes a favorite for a lot of people.

For binding loaves or burgers, try mashed potato, cooked oatmeal, fine bread crumbs, or tomato paste. For baking recipes that call for an egg or two, just leave them out, adding a little extra water for moisture. If a recipe calls for more than two eggs, use one of the following in place of each egg:

- ☞ an egg-sized piece of mashed banana, applesauce, puréed soft tofu, or canned pumpkin
- ☞ 1 tablespoon flaxseeds with ¼ cup water, puréed in a blender
- ☞ 1 tablespoon soy flour mixed with 2 tablespoons water
- ☞ 2 tablespoons cornstarch
- ☞ commercial egg replacers, available at natural food stores

Keep your eyes open for new possibilities. You'll find endless new flavors at international restaurants, grocery stores, and natural food stores. You can also find great ideas at the website of the Physicians Committee for Responsible Medicine (pcrm.org) and the many websites now devoted to vegan foods.

In the next chapter, we'll see how to tailor your menu to address specific health targets.

CHAPTER 4

Special Health Targets

NOW YOU'VE GOT THE BASICS DOWN. BUT YOU MAY WANT TO GO a step further. If you have a specific health concern—weight you would like to lose, diabetes, high cholesterol, or something else—you can build extra power into your vegan eating plan. In this chapter, I'll show you how.

Losing Weight

If you are trying to lose weight, going vegan will help enormously.[1] For starters, there is no longer even a drop of animal fat on your plate. That's great, because *every gram of fat holds 9 calories.* That's a lot more than are in carbohydrates or protein (just 4 calories per gram). To take an example, white-meat chicken—even without the skin—is about one-quarter fat, as a percentage of calories. In contrast, nearly all foods from plant sources—beans, grains, vegetables, and fruits— derive less than 10 percent of their calories from fat. So if you are skipping animal products and building your meals from plants, you're skipping a lot of unwanted calories.

FATTY FOODS PACK IN THE CALORIES

1 gram of carbohydrate, sugar, or protein = 4 calories

1 gram of fat = 9 calories

There are a few fatty foods in the plant world that you will want to be cautious about: vegetable oils, nuts, seeds, and avocados pack a fair amount of fat. Yes, their natural plant oils are much healthier than animal fats (most animal fats are high in the *saturated* fat that raises cholesterol levels and is linked to Alzheimer's disease, while most plant-derived oils have very little saturated fat). Even so, *all fats and oils have 9 calories in every gram.* So if weight loss is your goal, it's good not just to avoid animal products, but also to minimize oily foods, such as nuts, peanut butter, guacamole, and oils used in cooking. You will soon see what a difference this step can make.

What's a good goal? If you are aiming for weight loss, a total of 20 to 30 grams of fat in a day's meals is a good limit. That is much less than what most people get. But it is easily achieved when you're skipping animal products and limiting fatty foods.

If you are tracking your fat intake, fruits, vegetables, and other foods in the produce aisle do not have nutrition labels, so don't worry about them. For packaged foods, favor those that have no more than 2 to 3 grams of fat per serving. You'll see that, over the course of the day, you'll stay under your fat limit.

CUT THE FAT

In addition to avoiding animal products, here are some easy ways to cut the fat and all the calories that go with it.

- Instead of frying in oil, try sautéing in water, in vegetable broth, or even in a dry pan (e.g., for onions or garlic). Or use just a spritz of cooking spray or a nonstick pan.
- Skip nuts and nut butters. Yes, peanut butter and roasted almonds are tasty, but they are very high in fat calories.
- Top salads with nonfat dressing, lemon juice, balsamic vinegar, horseradish, or seasoned rice vinegar instead of oily dressings.
- On a sandwich, use mustard or pickle relish instead of mayonnaise. A squirt of seasoned vinegar works great on a sub.
- On toast, there is no need for butter or margarine if you've bought a good-quality bread.
- Top baked potatoes with black pepper, mustard, or salsa instead of butter.

Fiber: Your Weight-Loss Friend

For powering weight loss, it also pays to think about fiber—that is, plant roughage. Yes, "fiber" is a boring word from nutritional science. But it really does pack health power. Here's why: Fiber is filling but has essentially no calories. So although you might imagine you have eaten quite a lot, the truth is that fiber reins in your appetite and keeps your calorie intake in bounds. With high-fiber foods on your plate, you will push away from the table before you have overeaten.

Animal products have no fiber at all—zero—which is another reason why meaty, cheesy diets tend to fatten people up. But every bite of vegetables, fruit, beans, and whole grains includes fiber. At the top of the list is our humble friend the bean. Check out the numbers:

Fiber in Common Foods (in Grams)

Black beans (½ cup)	6
Baked beans (½ cup)	5
Broccoli (1 cup)	5
Apple (1 medium)	4
Brown rice (1 cup)	4
Oatmeal, cooked (1 cup)	4
Orange (1 medium)	3
Banana (1 medium)	3
Whole-grain cereal (1 cup)	3
White rice (1 cup)	2
Whole-grain breads (1 slice)	2
White bread or bagel (1 slice)	1
Spaghetti, cooked (½ cup)	0.5

Notice that, although whole-grain cereals brag about their fiber, the real fiber champs are beans and vegetables. And whole grains are better than refined grains. Notice what happens when brown rice sheds its bran coating to become white rice. It loses half of its fiber. That is also the case when you compare white bread to whole-grain breads. So, to power your weight loss, you'll want to put beans, vegetables, and fruits front and center in your routine, and favor whole grains over refined grains.

Simple, isn't it? By avoiding animal products, keeping oils low, and emphasizing high-fiber foods, you can make your weight loss easy—even without counting calories or saying no to seconds. These foods are naturally modest in calories, and they satisfy your brain's natural satiety mechanism so that your appetite turns off. Our research also found that a vegan diet gently boosts your metabolism in the after-meal period.[2] In other words, after people have been following a vegan diet for a few weeks, their bodies are better able to turn calories into body heat, rather than storing them as fat. The effect is small—your after-meal metabolism increases about 16 percent. But considering that the effect lasts three or more hours after each meal, it adds up to a helpful extra calorie burn.

➤ What about exercise? It helps, too, but modestly so. Running full tilt for two miles burns fewer calories than are in a 20-ounce soda. So exercise *in addition to* eating a healthy vegan diet, not instead of it. ◆

Extra Weight-Loss Power

- Avoid all animal products
- Keep oily foods (vegetable oils, fried foods, nuts, seeds, avocados) to a minimum
- Boost high-fiber foods

Lowering Cholesterol

Animal products drive cholesterol levels skyward. First of all, meat, dairy products, and eggs contain cholesterol—with eggs at the top of the list—and roughly half of the cholesterol you eat ends up in your bloodstream. Much worse is the *saturated* ("bad") fat in dairy products, meat, and eggs. It stimulates your body to make extra cholesterol.

Plants are just the opposite. They have very little saturated fat and are essentially cholesterol-free. So simply going vegan typically makes cholesterol levels fall sharply. If you like, you can boost your cholesterol-cutting power even more. Using a plant-based diet plus the "special effect foods" in the box on page 31, University of Toronto researchers lowered low-density lipoprotein (LDL, or "bad") cholesterol levels by nearly 30 percent *in just four weeks*.[3]

You don't need a lot of these foods. Just start with a vegan diet and include a serving of oats, barley, or beans, plus a soy product each day. If you add almonds, limit your intake to just an ounce (a small handful) a day. And cholesterol-lowering margarines are strictly optional.

Special Cholesterol-Lowering Foods

- Soluble fiber: oats, barley, or beans (a serving is 1 cup of cooked oats or barley or ½ cup of beans)
- Soy protein: soy milk, tofu, and soy meat substitutes (a serving is 1 cup of soy milk or 3 ounces of tofu)
- Almonds (a serving is 1 ounce)
- Special cholesterol-cutting margarines: e.g., Benecol (a serving is 2 teaspoons)

One other point: Although almost all plant foods are very low in saturated ("bad") fat, two big exceptions are coconut oil and palm oil. They are loaded with it. And even though they are added to many snack foods and other products for their buttery mouthfeel, they will raise your cholesterol (*and* pad your waistline), and you should skip them. Check the package label if you're buying prepared foods.

Tackling Diabetes

One of the most exciting breakthroughs in recent years is the discovery that type 2 diabetes is a two-way street. It can improve and sometimes even go away. Our research team has been studying diabetes for many years, and we have found that, although a conventional "diabetes diet" that focuses on cutting calories and counting

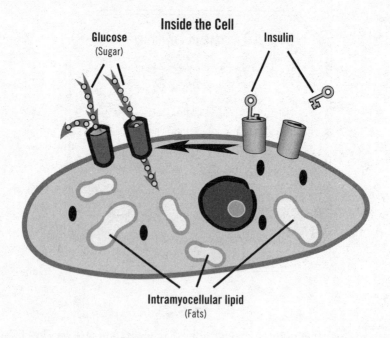

Inside the Cell

Glucose
(Sugar)

Insulin

Intramyocellular lipid
(Fats)

carbohydrate grams has only a limited benefit, a more powerful regimen brings more powerful results.

To see how this works, let's first understand what causes diabetes. Many people imagine that diabetes comes from eating sugar. That is certainly an understandable idea. After all, blood sugar levels are high in diabetes, so one might think that eating sugar somehow triggers the disease process. Many doctors and dietitians believed that, too, and they put diabetic patients on diets that limited sugar and carbohydrate-rich foods, such as rice and bread, because carbohydrates release sugar as they digest. They also cut calories, hoping to starve the weight off. But these methods have not helped very much. None of them make the disease go away. Most patients still need to start medication; then they need a second medication and a third, and before long they are on insulin injections in ever-increasing doses.

A revolutionary view of diabetes came from a look inside the muscle cells. Using high-tech scanning technology, researchers found that people with type 2 diabetes have particles of fat inside their muscle cells. That fat comes from foods, for the most part. And the fat buildup inside the cells makes it harder for sugar to pass from the bloodstream into the cells. More specifically, these fat particles interfere with insulin, the hormone that normally escorts sugar (glucose) from the bloodstream into the cells. Looking at the liver, the researchers found the same thing: Fat buildup in the liver cells meant that they could no longer remove sugar from the bloodstream normally.

Insulin is like a key. It attaches to receptors on the surface of the muscle and liver cells, like a key in a lock. Once the insulin "key" attaches to the receptor, it signals the cell to let in glucose. In type 2 diabetes that signaling process is not working and the culprit is fat buildup inside the cell.

As an analogy, imagine what would happen if a prankster put chewing gum into your front-door lock. Your key would no longer work. Fat buildup in your muscle and liver cells is a bit like that. It makes your insulin "key" malfunction. So, even though your natural insulin continues to attach to the receptors on each cell, it has more trouble opening the channels that allow glucose to come into the cell. Scientists call this fat buildup in muscle cells *intramyocellular lipid*.

That shows us the answer to the problem. If fat buildup in muscle cells and liver cells causes blood sugar levels to rise, the solution ought to be a low-fat vegan diet. After all, a vegan diet has no animal fat at all, and if vegetable oils are kept to a minimum, there is very little of any kind of fat. So that fat buildup in muscle and liver cells ought to start to dissipate. As I mentioned in Chapter 1, my research team was funded by the US government to do a head-to-head comparison of a low-fat vegan diet and a conventional diet that limited calories and carbohydrates. We found that a low-fat vegan diet is much more effective at controlling blood glucose levels.[4]

If you would like to try this for yourself, here is how to do it: Begin with the weight-loss steps mentioned at the beginning of this chapter (even if your weight is in the healthy range). That means, first, a vegan diet and, second, keeping added fats to a minimum. So skip the added oils and oily foods and the nuts and avocados, and favor high-fiber foods.

Then add one more step: When you choose breads or other carbohydrate-containing foods, pick those with the least effect on your blood sugar. These are foods with a low *Glycemic Index*. Here's how:

- ☞ Instead of added sugars, have fruit. Yes, fruit is sweet, but it has much less of an effect on your blood sugar compared with sugar itself.
- ☞ Instead of white and wheat breads, choose rye or pumpernickel.
- ☞ Instead of white baking potatoes, have sweet potatoes.
- ☞ Instead of typical cold cereals, have oatmeal or bran cereal.

You will find more details at glycemicindex.com.

Extra Power Against Diabetes

The three steps for tackling diabetes are:

- Avoid animal products.
- Keep oils and oily foods to a minimum.
- Favor low-Glycemic-Index foods.

If you have diabetes, it is essential to talk with your doctor or caregiver before making a diet change and to stay in touch as you begin, because a low-fat vegan diet can reduce your blood sugar quickly and powerfully. So if you are also taking medications, especially insulin, your blood sugar can even drop *too low*, to the point of being dangerous. Speak to your caregiver so he or she can reduce your medicines when the time is right. For more details, have a look at *Dr. Neal Barnard's Program for Reversing Diabetes*.

Improving Blood Pressure

Keeping blood pressure in a healthy range protects your heart, your kidneys, your brain, and all the rest of you. If you can do that without medications, you will skip their side effects and expense. In research studies, vegan diets consistently improve blood pressure.[5] They do that in three ways:

1. First, the saturated fat in dairy and meat products makes blood "thicker" (more viscous) and makes the artery walls stiffer, so it takes more pressure to move blood through the arteries. A vegan diet reduces blood viscosity and makes arteries more flexible, improving blood flow.

2. Second, plants are naturally low in sodium (which raises blood pressure) and rich in potassium (which lowers it). Contrast that with dairy products, especially cheese, which is loaded with sodium. Because many canned soups, other canned products, and snacks have added salt, you will want to favor low-sodium brands.

3. Third, losing unwanted weight brings blood pressure down. As a vegan diet naturally helps your body shed unwanted pounds, you will see your blood pressure improve more and more as the weight comes off.

So the first two factors (the improvement in blood viscosity and the preference for potassium over sodium) will bring down blood pressure fairly quickly, and weight loss adds to the improvement gradually as the pounds melt away. If you add exercise, you'll lower your blood pressure even more.

Once again, let your caregiver know you are changing your diet, so that your medications can be reduced when the time is right. Do not adjust them on your own. And if these steps have not lowered your blood pressure to the healthy range, follow your doctor's advice about medication.

Extra Power for Lowering Blood Pressure

- Avoid animal products and added oils.
- Keep salt intake modest. Read labels and stay under 1,500 milligrams of sodium per day.
- Add regular exercise.

Preventing Cancer

A plant-based diet is a powerful way to reduce cancer risk. For people who have been diagnosed with cancer, it is an important way to improve survival. The reasons are not hard to find.

☞ As chicken or other meats are cooked, carcinogens called *heterocyclic amines* form within the muscle tissue. That can happen when meats are fried, baked, or heated in any other way. And grilling produces additional carcinogens. In turn, these carcinogens can alter your DNA, turning a normal cell into a cancer cell.

☞ Meats also alter the gut bacteria so that they are more likely to produce carcinogens in your intestinal tract.

☞ Dairy products have been linked to prostate cancer.[6] Part of the problem is that milk increases a compound in the bloodstream called IGF-1 (insulin-like growth factor), which stimulates cancer cell growth. In addition, as the calcium in milk floods into your bloodstream, your body reacts to limit the influx of calcium to a safe level. To do that, it reduces the amount of vitamin D in your blood (vitamin D helps the body to absorb calcium). But because vitamin D also has cancer-preventive effects, this loss of vitamin D increases cancer risk. At least, that is the theory. Men who avoid milk, cheese, and other dairy have been shown to have substantially less risk, compared with their milk-drinking friends.

Avoiding animal products allows you to sidestep these risks. And plants have specific anticancer effects.

+>===+==<+

Extra Power to Prevent Cancer

- Vegetables and fruits are rich in cancer-fighting micronutrients, including folate (think green leafy vegetables), vitamin C (citrus fruit), beta-carotene (orange vegetables), and lycopene (tomatoes and watermelon), among many others.
- Cruciferous vegetables (e.g., broccoli, Brussels sprouts, cabbage, kale, cauliflower, and their cousins) stimulate the liver to make enzymes that neutralize carcinogens that you may be exposed to.
- Fiber, which is abundant in foods from plants but absent from animal products, helps prevent colorectal cancer and also helps remove excess hormones that could otherwise contribute to cancer of the breast, prostate, and other hormone-sensitive organs.

A cancer-prevention diet skips animal products and emphasizes healthful vegetables, fruits, beans, and whole grains in as natural (unprocessed) a form as possible. The weight-control steps outlined earlier in this chapter are helpful, too; a trimmer waistline reduces the risk of several forms of cancer.

➤ Red wine may be in the "fruit group," so to speak, but alcohol in any form increases the risk of breast cancer, colon cancer, and other forms of the disease. ◀

Cancer Survival

Foods do more than reduce the likelihood that cancer will strike. For people with cancer, foods can improve survival. Although more research on the effects of foods on cancer survival is needed, certain keys have emerged. For women diagnosed with breast cancer, it pays to avoid excess fats and to emphasize fruits and vegetables.[7,8] Adding exercise appears to be helpful, too. For men diagnosed with prostate cancer, a low-fat vegan diet has been shown to improve survival.[9] Similar diet changes may help with survival from colorectal cancer. There is less information on how foods affect other forms of the disease.

Soy products reduce the risk of developing breast cancer and improve survival in women previously diagnosed with breast cancer.

That's right. While some people have raised the question as to whether soy products might increase cancer risk, studies have shown precisely the opposite; they have a beneficial cancer-preventing effect.

The biological explanation for this benefit is not entirely clear. However, women who consume the most soy (soy milk, tofu, etc.) have about 30 to 40 percent less risk of developing breast cancer,[10,11] and those previously diagnosed with cancer are about 30 percent less likely to die of their cancer, compared with their soy-avoiding friends.[12]

Protecting Your Brain

In 2003, Chicago researchers reported a stunning finding: People who generally avoided "bad" fats dramatically reduced their risk of developing Alzheimer's disease.[13] In this case, "bad" fats mean two things: the *saturated* fat (solid fat) found in dairy products and meat and the *trans* fats (partially hydrogenated oils) found in snack foods. So a vegan diet is a great start because it avoids most of the saturated fats. And kicking out pastries or fried snacks that include partially hydrogenated oils (you'll see them on the label) is a good idea, too.

There are extra steps you can take:

Avoid Harmful Metals

Although your body needs traces of iron and copper, they are harmful in excess. In the same way that iron rusts and a copper penny gradually darkens, these metals can oxidize *in your body*, triggering the production of *free radicals*—dangerous molecules that can damage the brain. Aluminum, too: Evidence suggests that it can be toxic to the brain. A vegan diet helps you avoid the iron overload that can come from meat and liver.

⊷⊷

> ➤ **It also pays to avoid cookware that puts iron, copper, or aluminum directly in contact with food. Yes, that old favorite cast-iron pan may actually be part of the problem if you are using it every day. (Stainless steel is okay, as is nonstick cookware, provided the layer under the nonstick coating is steel.)** ⊱

⊷⊷

Avoid multivitamins that contain iron and copper, and steer clear of aluminum-containing antacids. When selecting a deodorant, look for those that omit aluminum, as it can pass through the skin into the blood.

☞ **Get your vitamin E.** Vitamin E–rich foods reduce Alzheimer's risk. That means almonds, walnuts, sunflower seeds, pecans, pine nuts, pistachios, sesame seeds, and flaxseed. Go easy, because these are fatty, high-calorie foods. Just one small handful of nuts or seeds a day is plenty.

☞ **Eat for color.** Some evidence suggests that grapes, blueberries, and other brightly colored berries can improve memory in older people with mild memory problems. Their color comes from *anthocyanins*, which are powerful antioxidants that can knock out free radicals.

☞ **Lace up your sneakers.** A University of Illinois study showed that a forty-minute brisk walk three times a week improves memory and reverses brain shrinkage.[14]

☞ **Get plenty of sleep.** Don't forget to rest! Getting adequate sleep is essential for brain health. Sleep is when the brain files away the events of the day, integrating them into your memory reserves. During sleep, your brain also restores your emotional stability. Without it, your memory and emotional control will be less than optimal. Everyone's needs are different, but eight hours a night is a good goal.

Stopping Inflammation and Pain

For inflammatory conditions, such as rheumatoid arthritis, a surprising culprit could be animal *protein*. To understand how, let's take an analogy. Let's say you accidentally get a splinter. The splinter triggers inflammation in your skin; that is your skin's natural response to injury or invasion. Your blood vessels open up to bring blood flow to the region, so the area looks red, and the influx of blood and fluid causes swelling. Blood flow brings white blood cells to the region, and each blood cell is like a little Pac-Man trying to gobble up the splinter particles that don't belong there.

Inflammation is caused not just by splinters but also by certain foods. Among the chief suspects are dairy proteins. Several different research teams have found that people with arthritis do much better when they set aside dairy products, particularly as part of a vegan diet. This is especially true of *rheumatoid* arthritis but may also be true of other forms of the disease, as well as other conditions, including migraine.

So if you have an inflammatory condition, it makes good sense to start a vegan diet, and to do it 100 percent, because even small amounts of problem foods can trigger inflammation.

➤ If avoiding animal products does not fully resolve the problem, it is possible that you have more than one trigger. For example, some people might be affected by dairy products, in addition to eggs, wheat, or tomatoes—or perhaps by citrus fruits and nuts. So, to track down your trigger foods, you can try a simple elimination diet that removes all the potential food triggers and then reintroduces them one at a time, so you can see which ones cause problems. The details are in my prior books *The Cheese Trap* and *Foods That Fight Pain*. ◄

Athletic Power and Endurance

Vegan diets have tremendous benefits for athletes. If you want to optimize your performance, whether in a game or in your workouts, cutting out animal products is one of the most effective ways to do that.

First, the anti-inflammatory steps described in the previous section help cut post-workout recovery times, so athletes are ready to get back in the game much sooner.

Second, vegan foods boost endurance. As we saw in the discussion of high blood pressure, plant-based diets make the blood "thinner," that is, less viscous. That does not just reduce blood pressure. It also increases the oxygenation of the muscles and brain. That's part of why vegan diets give athletes better endurance.

Third, plants are packed with healthful complex carbohydrates to build *glycogen*. Glycogen is a special form of glucose that your liver and muscles store for extra energy, like spare batteries. If you have heard of athletes "carbo-loading," this is what they are talking about. They are eating plenty of rice, bread, pasta, sweet potatoes, and other healthy carbohydrate-rich foods in order to store extra glycogen in their muscles and liver for long-lasting power.

As you can see, a vegan diet provides extraordinary power for tackling health conditions. More details on using foods to tackle health problems are available in the Recommended Resources listed on pages 101–5.

CHAPTER 5

Complete Nutrition

SOME PEOPLE WONDER IF A VEGAN DIET WILL GIVE THEM all the nutrition they need. Actually, a plant-based diet provides *better* nutrition than a diet including meat and dairy products. Harvard researchers developed a system for rating the healthfulness of various eating patterns, called the *Alternate Healthy Eating Index*. It turns out that vegan diets score much better than diets including meat and dairy products. Surprised? Well, meat is low in many vitamins and minerals. It has no vitamin C and no fiber at all, and it is high in saturated ("bad") fat and cholesterol. Yes, meat does have protein and iron, but so do plants, in more healthful forms. Similarly, dairy products have lots of fat, protein, and sugar and miss the vitamins that are in vegetables, fruits, and beans.

In our research studies, we track what happens when people adopt plant-based diets. Good news: Their nutrition improves dramatically.[15] Plant-based foods provide the right amount of protein, a better quality of fat, abundant healthful carbohydrates for energy, fiber for healthy digestion and cancer prevention, and vitamins and minerals in far better proportions than are found in animal products.

Even so, you might be wondering about getting adequate protein, calcium, and other nutrients. So let's take a quick look at the details.

Okay, So Where Do You Get Your Protein?

According to the US government, women need about 46 grams of protein per day. Men need about 56 grams. The actual amounts needed are likely less; these numbers include a margin for safety.

If you were to eat nothing but broccoli for a day, you would get 146 grams of protein on a typical 2,000-calorie diet. The next day, if you were to eat nothing but lentils, you would get 157 grams of protein. Pinto beans? 186 grams. If you were to eat only oatmeal, you would get 62 grams of pure protein. Of course, I'm not suggesting that you actually eat just one food in a day—this is just an illustration—but the point is that plants have *lots* of protein. You are probably aware that there is a lot of protein in soy products; true enough, but vegetables and grains have protein, too.

Protein in Everyday Foods

(Grams of protein in 2,000 calories)

Pinto beans	186
Lentils	157
Broccoli	146
Peas	135
Corn	79
Oatmeal	62
Carrots	49
Blueberries	48
Brown rice	43
Potatoes (skinless)	42

So, plants have protein. "But is it *complete* protein?" you may ask. Proteins are actually long chains of *amino acids*, joined together like beads on a necklace. *Complete* protein is protein that has all the amino acids you need. Decades ago, some people imagined that one had to carefully combine various plants to get "complete protein." But it turns out that any normal variety of plant-based foods brings you all the amino acids you need. In its official position paper, the Academy of Nutrition and Dietetics says, "Protein needs at all ages, including those for athletes, are well achieved by balanced vegetarian diets."[16]

Calcium Straight from the Source

Where do you get calcium without dairy products? Well, cows don't actually make calcium at all. Calcium comes from the Earth. Green vegetables pull calcium from the soil through their roots, and it ends up in their leaves. When cows eat grass, calcium passes into their milk. You can get the calcium you need directly from plants, too—hopefully not grass! But there is abundant calcium in broccoli, Brussels sprouts, kale, collards, and other green leafy vegetables. In fact, their calcium is actually more absorbable than that in milk. An exception is spinach, which is a rather selfish vegetable; it will not release much of its calcium. But most green vegetables provide plenty of highly absorbable calcium. It pays to emphasize them in your routine. Beans provide calcium, too, as do squash, sweet potatoes, tofu, figs, oranges, and raisins, among many other foods. If you are looking for extra calcium, calcium-fortified nondairy milks (e.g., calcium-fortified soy milk, almond milk, and rice milk) are loaded with it.

Calcium (milligrams per 1-cup serving)

Collards: 357

Tofu, firm: 355

Kale: 180

Figs, dried: 149

Butternut squash: 84

Raisins: 82

Chickpeas: 80

Pinto beans: 79

Sweet potatoes: 76

Oranges: 71

Broccoli: 62

Brussels sprouts: 56

Iron, the Healthy Way

You need iron to make the hemoglobin that your blood cells use to transport oxygen, and the best sources are green leafy vegetables and beans. In fact, in our research studies, people adopting a vegan diet often get slightly *more* iron than they did on a meat-and-dairy diet, thanks to the iron in greens and beans.

In the 1950s, the idea was "the more iron, the better." Television shows advertised the iron supplement Geritol as the answer to "tired blood." But soon it became clear that extra iron is dangerous. If there is too much iron in your body, it can spark the production of dangerous *free radicals*, which can harm the heart and brain and contribute to the aging process. So while the body needs a trace of iron, overdoing it is risky.

Plants have a healthful form of iron, called *nonheme* iron, that is *more absorbable when your body is low in iron and less absorbable when your body already has plenty on board.* That way, you get the iron you need without overdosing. Meat has a form of iron called *heme* iron, which is highly absorbed whether you need it or not. That can lead to iron overload.

Bottom line: Greens and beans have the iron you need in the healthiest possible form.

> **Iron (milligrams per 1-cup serving):**
>
> Chickpeas: 4.7
>
> Pinto beans: 3.6
>
> Raisins: 3.1
>
> Kale: 1.2
>
> Broccoli: 1.1
>
> Sweet potatoes: 1.0

Vitamin B_{12}: Easy, but Essential

Vitamin B_{12} is essential for healthy nerves and healthy blood cells. But it is not made by plants or animals. It is made by bacteria. Some people speculate that, before the advent of modern hygiene, the traces of bacteria in the soil, on vegetables, on our fingers, and in our mouths gave us the traces of B_{12} we needed. Whether that is true or not, modern hygiene has eliminated that possibility.

Meat and dairy products contain traces of B_{12} because an animal's intestinal tract harbors bacteria that produce it. But those are hardly healthful sources because along with it come cholesterol, "bad" fat, and other problems. In addition, many people have trouble absorbing B_{12} from animal products. Many older people do not produce enough stomach acid to separate the B_{12} from the protein it is bound to, and common medications (e.g., metformin, often used to treat type 2 diabetes, and acid blockers) interfere with its absorption. So, even while eating animal products, they do not absorb adequate B_{12}. A vegan diet, of course, does not include meat or dairy products.

The simplest thing to do is to take a vitamin B_{12} supplement. Every drugstore and natural food store sells them. Adults need 2.4 micrograms per day, according to the US government, and all common brands have more than that (some have much more). So pick up any common brand with a modest dose (e.g., 50 micrograms) and take it daily. You will see it in two forms, cyanocobalamin and methylcobalamin. Both are effective.

➤◄

➤ On a vegan diet, it is essential to add a source of B_{12}. Don't skip this. A B_{12} deficiency can take years to develop, but the first sign can be nerve symptoms that are irreversible. ◄

Vitamin D

Vitamin D is produced by sunlight on your skin. It helps you absorb calcium from the foods you eat and also helps protect against cancer. About twenty minutes of sunlight on your face and arms a few times each week gives you the vitamin D you need. But if you are not getting regular sun exposure, or if you use a sunscreen, a vitamin D supplement can be very helpful. A daily dose of 2,000 international units is considered safe.

Do I Really Need to Take Supplements?

Some people resist taking a supplement of vitamin B_{12} or D because "nature ought to provide the nutrition we need." True enough. But you don't live in nature. You live in New Jersey. Or maybe Portland or Glasgow or Reykjavík or Oslo or Tierra del Fuego or somewhere else where there is not enough sunlight, in all likelihood. Had our forebears had the good judgment to remain in sunny eastern Africa, we would have gotten all the vitamin D anyone could ever want.

Similarly, it may well be that in our less-than-hygienic past, bacterially produced B_{12} was more abundant than it is today. It's also possible that when we ate more healthfully, we were able to absorb the B_{12} produced by our own gut bacteria. Who knows? But because humans have moved away from nature, supplements of vitamin B_{12} and (for those not getting regular sunlight) vitamin D play important roles.

Omega-3s

Although some fats are risky—saturated fats raise cholesterol, for example—your body does need traces of good fats. One in particular is called *ALA*, or *alpha-linolenic acid*. The name is not important, though what is important is that it is a healthful omega-3 fatty acid that your body will lengthen into another omega-3, called DHA (docosahexaenoic acid), that your brain uses. Where do you find it? There are ALA traces in green leafy vegetables, fruits, and beans, and much larger amounts in walnuts and various seeds. If these foods are in your routine, you'll get the healthy fats your body needs.

Some people use omega-3 supplements. Some of these supplements are vegan; others come from fish oil. Their benefit has not yet been proven. A potential disadvantage of these products is that they can make bleeding more of a problem. That is, they make it harder to stop bleeding when you have a cut or have surgery, and internal bleeding may be more likely. So my suggestion is to take advantage of the traces of healthful fats in green leafy vegetables, fruits, and beans and to minimize the use of competing fats and oils. Hopefully, further research will clarify what, if any, role there may be for omega-3 supplements.

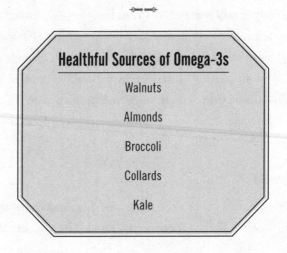

Healthful Sources of Omega-3s

Walnuts

Almonds

Broccoli

Collards

Kale

A vegan diet that relies primarily on whole foods will naturally give you great nutrition. Everyone also needs vitamin B_{12}, and if you're not getting sunlight, you'll need a vitamin D supplement, too. But that is about it. It pays to favor green leafy vegetables for calcium. For most people, there is no need for a multivitamin or other vitamin supplements (unless your caregiver has specifically called for them). You'll get the nutrition you need from food.

CHAPTER 6

Vegan for Every Life Stage

A VEGAN DIET IS GREAT AT EVERY STAGE OF LIFE. THERE ARE a few things to think about at various points along the way, and this chapter will provide some important tips that let you take advantage of vegan power during pregnancy, breastfeeding, infancy, childhood, and older age.

Vegan Foods During Pregnancy

At what age can children start a vegan diet? The answer is at conception. A plant-based diet is great for a developing baby, and it's great for Mom, too. Women who stick to vegan diets during pregnancy may have fewer complications, compared with omnivores. For example, a condition called *preeclampsia* occurs in 3 to 4 percent of pregnancies, manifesting as a dangerous rise in blood pressure. Decades ago, researchers studied the medical records of vegan mothers, finding preeclampsia to be much less common in this group. They found only 1 case in 775 pregnancies—as opposed to the usual 1 in 25.[17]

Unfortunately, pregnant women are the recipients of abundant unsolicited advice on what they should be eating, and it can be hard to know what advice is worth listening to. So let's look at the basics.

How Much to Eat?

You will no doubt be reminded that you are "eating for two." True enough, but one of you is very small. So the increased nutrition you require is modest. According to the Academy of Nutrition and Dietetics, it works out to about 340 extra calories each day in the second trimester (that's the equivalent of an extra cup of rice and an apple each day) and about 450 extra calories during the third (the rice and apple, plus a banana).[18] There is no need to add extra high-protein foods to the menu; extra servings of vegetables, beans, and grains bring protein along with them. And there is never a need for meat, fish, dairy products, or other animal-derived products.

Foods for a Healthy Pregnancy

The best nutrition comes from our familiar four staples—vegetables, fruits, whole grains, and legumes (beans, peas, and lentils), plus your prenatal vitamins.

Skip dairy products. Your most healthful calcium sources, as we saw earlier, are "greens and beans." There are plenty of other sources, too, as we saw in Chapter 5. You will want to emphasize them in your routine. You do not need dairy products at all, and I would encourage you to avoid them. Here is why.

First of all, dairy products are one of the leading suspects as a cause of type 1 diabetes. The theory is that dairy proteins trigger the production of antibodies in the baby's body that can destroy the insulin-producing cells of the pancreas. This theory is still under investigation, but researchers have long known three things that would suggest there's something to this: First, certain dairy proteins can pass into your bloodstream; second, children diagnosed with type 1 diabetes have antibodies to cow's milk proteins circulating in their bloodstream, and they are found at much higher concentrations than in children who do not develop diabetes. These antibodies may well have been the ones that destroyed their insulin-producing cells. Third, children who are never exposed to cow's milk have less risk of developing type 1 diabetes. Since we do not know the age of greatest vulnerability to developing diabetes—before birth, during infancy, or in early childhood—I suggest that pregnant or breastfeeding women avoid dairy products entirely and avoid giving them to their children as well.

Skip meat. While we tend to think of the risks of fat and cholesterol—or of unhealthy foods in general—as applying only to older people, it pays to protect your developing baby, too. Meat products have fat, cholesterol, and a load of unnecessary calories, making meat-eaters significantly heavier than people who avoid meat. Excess weight gain in pregnancy can pose risks to your baby. Some particularly chilling findings recently emerged in a study of twenty-three women and their newborns at the University of Sydney, in Australia. Researchers measured the thickness of the babies' blood vessel walls, which can be done easily and noninvasively. It turned out that babies born to overweight mothers had thicker aortic walls. In other words, for these babies, *heart disease had begun in utero.* These infants are also more likely to show signs of inflammation at birth, measured using a test called C-reactive protein, or CRP.[19] In other words, mothers' unhealthy diets were apparently triggering disease processes in their infants before birth. They are set up for a lifetime of weight problems and for increased risk of damage to their hearts and blood vessels. While heart disease and artery damage are, to an extent, reversible, the best time to stop them is before they start. That means a healthful, well-planned, plant-based diet from day one.

> ➢ **Pregnancy is also a great time to be glad you are not eating fish. As you know, mercury and other pollutants end up in many fish species, and they can easily reach your developing baby. With a vegan diet, you're skipping them all.** ➢

Know Your Prenatal Vitamins

While there are shelves filled with vitamins at stores, the simplest thing is to take a basic prenatal vitamin. Vegan prenatal vitamins (including iron-free brands) are widely available. You will find them at natural food stores and online.

And if you can, it pays to start *before* you become pregnant. Prenatal vitamins contain folic acid, which protects against neurological deficits that can occur within the first few weeks of fetal development.

Prenatal vitamins also include vitamin B_{12}, which you already know is essential at all stages of life. And rather than having a whopping B_{12} dose every several days, as some people do (simply because some common B_{12} brands are so large), it's better to have a small dose on a daily basis, so prenatal vitamins have you covered.

It also helps to make sure your vitamin is providing you with vitamin D, which as we've discussed helps your body absorb calcium from the foods you eat. Normally, it is produced by sunlight on your skin, as you know. Hopefully you are getting out in the sun regularly. But because many people do not get much sun exposure, especially in the winter months, prenatal vitamins include vitamin D. They also have calcium, which is important for bone development.

A word about iron: There is abundant iron in green leafy vege-tables and beans, and iron absorption is improved when you have vitamin C–rich foods along with it (e.g., those orange slices in your salad). Most prenatal vitamins include iron. Unfortunately, iron supplements can sometimes aggravate nausea or constipation. And, over your life span, excess iron can actually be harmful in other ways, increasing the risk of heart problems and possibly even Alzheimer's disease. Since many women get plenty of iron in food, some experts advocate skipping iron supplementation early in pregnancy and giving it in the second or third trimesters only if blood tests show you need it. That said, women who are not having their iron status checked are better off taking prenatal vitamins with iron.

DHA. Some people recommend taking supplements of DHA during pregnancy. As we saw in Chapter 5, your body makes DHA from natural plant oils in the foods you eat. For example, broccoli, kale, walnuts, and almonds have traces of the natural oils your body needs. However, not everyone eats their greens and other healthful foods, and so not everyone has the right balance of natural oils in their diet, raising concern about whether they are able to make the DHA they need. That is where the question of DHA supplements comes in. Some authorities feel they may protect brain development. Unfortunately, the jury is still out as to whether DHA supplementation is beneficial, so we do not yet have clear guidance as to DHA supplements' value. Should you choose to take them, you can find vegan DHA (derived from algae) in health food stores and online.

What about alcohol? How much alcohol is safe during preg-nancy? The answer is zero. Not even a little bit at any point during pregnancy, including times when you are trying to get pregnant. If you are pregnant or might be pregnant, it is important to avoid alcohol.

Vegan Foods During Breastfeeding

Breastfeeding provides the best possible nourishment for babies, and a vegan diet gives you the nutrition you need to feed yourself and your baby. At first, breastfeeding can be awkward or even uncomfortable. This will pass. Let me encourage you to get advice from experienced family members, a lactation consultant, or La Leche League. You will be glad you did.

The guidelines for foods during pregnancy apply pretty well to breastfeeding, too: Focus on healthful vegetables, fruits, whole grains, and legumes. Don't forget your calcium-rich greens and beans. And be sure to have a source of vitamin B_{12}, which could mean continuing to take your prenatal vitamins or taking any common vitamin B_{12} supplement. You need B_{12} and so does your baby, who will get it from your breast milk, so don't skip it. If you are not getting regular sunlight, you will need a vitamin D supplement, too. Some people recommend DHA during breastfeeding—although the evidence remains uncertain—so the comments about DHA apply here, too.

Here's an important note: Some foods that you eat can make your baby colicky. In 1991, researchers found that intact cow's milk proteins can pass from a mother's digestive tract into her bloodstream and eventually into her breast milk, reaching her breastfeeding baby in sufficient quantity to upset the baby's stomach.[20] So if you have ice cream, cheese, or a glass of milk, tiny amounts of cow's milk protein can end up in your breast milk and can affect your child.

Other foods can do the same. Researchers have asked women which foods in their own diets seem to trigger colic in their breastfeeding babies. The problem foods seem to be cow's milk, coffee, chocolate, onions, and cruciferous vegetables (e.g., broccoli, cauliflower, and cabbage). So, as much as I love green leafy vegetables, if they are making your infant colicky, you'll want to turn to the other calcium-rich foods mentioned in Chapter 5.

Foods During Infancy

Babies should breastfeed for at least twelve months and can continue for two years or even longer. If breastfeeding is not possible, for whatever reason, soy-based baby formulas are a good alternative. Note that babies need baby *formula*, not the soy milk sold for drinking or splashing on your cereal.

By five or six months, babies are ready to add a bit of solid food. Iron-fortified warmed cereal is a good first choice, because by that point your baby has about used up the iron he or she got in the womb. Mix cereal with a little breast milk or soy formula.

➻ Hold off on wheat cereal until your baby is at least eight months old; it sometimes causes allergies. ❦

Other iron-rich foods include lentils, beet purée, blended spinach in a fruit smoothie, or hot mushy cereal with a splash of molasses. You'll want to introduce one new simple food at a time at one- to two-week intervals.

Foods at Six to Eight Months

At around six months, you can try slightly more adventurous foods:

☞ Vegetables—potatoes, green beans, carrots, and peas—all very well cooked and mashed

☞ Fruits, such as mashed bananas, avocados, strained peaches, and applesauce

At about eight months, breads, crackers, and dry cereal can be served. And your infant is now ready for higher-protein foods, such as very well-cooked mashed beans or tofu.

There is never a need for infants to have meat, dairy products, or eggs. As we have seen, these products create problems for them, just as they do later in life. Dairy products are a well-known cause of constipation in toddlers, leading to blood loss and other problems. The concerns raised about type 1 diabetes mentioned earlier apply here, too. I know that it can often be challenging to shield children from unhealthful foods, especially when you are on the go, at parties, and so forth. We'll have plenty of tips to help you in Chapter 8.

Foods for Growing Children

After the age of weaning, children's diets are not so different from those of adults and are built from our familiar healthful staples: vegetables, fruits, whole grains, and legumes. A few quick kid-friendly tips:

☞ **Stick to simple foods.** Most kids prefer simple foods, so corn, carrots, and green beans go over bigger than more complex tastes (e.g., grilled asparagus or marinated artichoke hearts), but give them a chance to see what they like.

☞ **Provide snacks.** Children are super active but have small stomachs, so healthful snacks, such as fresh fruit, soy milk, or crackers, come in handy.

☞ **Skip animal products.** Remember that artery disease begins in childhood. So kids should not have meat, dairy products, eggs, or unhealthful fats. And in case you were wondering, they do not need meat for normal growth.[21] As we saw in Chapter 5, it is easy to get complete nutrition from a vegan diet. Children thrive on healthful plant-based diets.

☞ **Try soy.** Soy products (veggie dogs, tofu) are fine. Some parents have heard that soy products contain "hormones" that could lead to breast cancer in girls or feminization in boys. The truth is just the opposite. Women who grew up with soy milk, tofu, or other soy products have *less* risk of developing cancer, and men who grew up with these same foods have no impairment of fertility, masculinity, athletic prowess, or anything else. And if they are labeled "organic," these products cannot be produced from genetically modified soybeans. You can find more details on this in Chapter 10.

☞ **Let them help.** Depending on their age, allowing children to help prepare the meal can greatly increase their interest in trying new foods. Even a tiny tot can help tear up lettuce. Getting them involved in food preparation will build their confidence, will help them develop motor skills, and may even let them tackle a few math problems.

☞ **Include nuts and seeds.** Although nuts, nut butters, and seeds are high in fat and calories, most authorities are more liberal with these foods for growing children than they would be for adults who are battling weight problems.

☞ **Supplement with vitamin B_{12}.** Nursing infants will get vitamin B_{12} from breast milk or formula. For older children, the recommended dietary allowance increases from 0.9 microgram in one-year-olds to 2.4 micrograms for fourteen-year-olds. Typical supplements and multivitamins contain this much or more, and B_{12} is essential for all children and adults.

Children who are raised on a healthful vegan diet have a huge measure of protection for their health. Their risk of heart disease, cancer, obesity, diabetes, and other conditions is cut dramatically. Children who never drink cow's milk have just as good bone development as children who do. And children who skip meat do as well as or better than their meat-eating friends. Vegan kids have normal growth and have a measure of protection against weight problems, diabetes, hypertension, asthma, and other health issues that are common in their not-yet-vegan friends.

Meal Planning for Kids—Made Simple

The following table shows the approximate numbers of daily servings that are appropriate for children as they grow. But these are rough estimates. Every child is different. Monitor your child's body weight and adjust the servings if needed.

A DAY'S MEALS
for a 2- to 3-Year-Old

BREAKFAST

Oatmeal: ½ cup cooked oats with 2 tablespoons raisins
made with 4 ounces soy milk

Water

SNACK

Apple: ½ sliced (skin removed for younger children)

LUNCH

Peanut butter and banana sandwich: 1 slice whole-grain bread,
2 tablespoons peanut butter, ¼ banana

Soy milk: 4 ounces

SNACK

Carrots and hummus: 2 tablespoons hummus and ½ cup carrot spears

DINNER

Beans and rice: ¼ cup cooked lentils and ½ cup cooked rice

½ cup roasted broccoli

⊷⊶

A DAY'S MEALS

for a 4- to 8-Year-Old

BREAKFAST

Almond butter toast: 2 slices whole-grain toast
with 2 tablespoons almond butter

Water

SNACK

Green smoothie: 1 cup spinach, 1 cup grapes, 1 cup soy milk, ½ pear

LUNCH

Bean tacos: 2 small flour or corn tortillas, ¼ cup black beans,
¼ cup rice, ¼ cup corn, ½ cup lettuce, 2 tablespoons salsa

Water

SNACK

Baked sweet potato sprinkled with cinnamon

Water

DINNER

Veggie stir-fry with tofu over noodles: 1 cup cooked pasta,
½ cup cooked tofu, 1 tablespoon sesame seeds,
½ cup carrots, ½ cup cabbage

Water

	2- to 3-year-olds	4- to 8-year-olds	What's a serving?
Fruit	1 serving	1.5 servings	1 cup fruit ½ cup raisins
Vegetables	1 serving	3 servings	1 cup vegetables
Legumes	2 servings	6 servings	1 Tbsp. nut butter ¼ cup cooked legumes 2 Tbsp. hummus ¼ cup cubed tofu
Grains	3 servings	2.5 servings	1 slice bread ½ cup cooked grain ½ cup cooked pasta
Dairy	2 servings	2.5 servings	1 cup soy milk

Before long, children will reach the age where they eat essentially like adults. For them, a healthy eating pattern will be based on the same healthful food groups, plus the supplement considerations we discussed in Chapter 2 and Chapter 5.

Adults at Older Ages

Older age is when many diet-related diseases—heart disease, diabetes, hypertension, and cancer—take their greatest toll, meaning that this is a time when a vegan diet is more important than ever. A few pointers:

Focus on vegetables. Dark green vegetables are rich in calcium for healthy bones, are important for cancer prevention, and provide micronutrients that help prevent macular degeneration, a common cause of visual impairment.

Feed your head. As we saw in Chapter 4, research shows that Alzheimer's disease is less common in people who avoid the *saturated* fat found in dairy products and meats and also avoid the trans fats found in some snack foods. There are other steps you can take to protect your brain, so have another look at Chapter 4.

Vitamins B_{12} and D. Older folks are at higher risk of vitamin B_{12} deficiency. That is because they make less stomach acid, which is needed to separate B_{12} from proteins, and many are on metformin (commonly used to treat type 2 diabetes), acid blockers, or other drugs that interfere with B_{12} absorption. This is another reason for B_{12} supplements. They are absorbable without stomach acid. And if you are missing out on daily sunlight, you'll want to supplement with vitamin D, too, as we saw in Chapter 5. If you are taking a multivitamin, choose one without added iron or copper.

Medications

➤ If you are on medications for diabetes, hypertension, or other conditions, talk with your health care provider as you change your diet, because your medication doses may need to be adjusted downward as you begin your new healthful food plan. Also, some medications are constipating, so high-fiber foods (beans, vegetables, fruits, and whole grains) are particularly important. ◀

If You Take a Blood Thinner.

If you take a blood thinner called *warfarin* (sold under the brand name Coumadin) to prevent blood clots that could lead to a stroke, heart attack, or other problems, you might have been told by your doctor that you need to avoid vegetables. What your doctor meant was that warfarin works by blocking vitamin K, which is involved in the clotting process. Because vegetables have vitamin K, your doctor is thinking that they will interfere with warfarin's anticlotting effect.

A better answer is not to avoid vegetables, but simply to keep the amount of vegetables you eat more or less steady from day to day. That way, your doctor can set your warfarin dose and keep it stable. And, of course, many prescribers are using newer blood thinners that do not raise this issue at all.

As we have seen, plant-based foods are great for every stage of life. In the next chapter, we will see how to make food preparation easy and quick.

CHAPTER 7

Make It Easy,
Make It Quick

W E'VE TALKED A LOT ABOUT WHY TO GO VEGAN, BUT LET'S discuss the all-important *how*. Feeling too pressed for time to cook? Have no inclination to become a gourmet chef? You are not alone! Luckily, meal preparation is easier than ever. Let's check out some shortcuts that will save you time. We'll also demystify the shopping experience.

Frozen Foods

Frozen foods are quick and convenient. Have a look at the freezer case in a natural food store or supermarket. Right next to the cheese-laden pizzas you will find vegan pizzas with all the taste and none of the regrets. You will also find vegan burritos, shepherd's pies, curries, and endless other dinners ready to pop in the oven or microwave.

While you are at the freezer case, pick up some precut broccoli, spinach, carrots, cauliflower, and Brussels sprouts. You can steam them in minutes, and their nutritional value is equivalent to that of fresh varieties.

Canned Foods

Canned soups, vegetables, and beans are convenient and quick. Low-sodium brands are widely available.

Salad Bars, Hot Food Bars

Many grocery stores feature hot and cold salad bars or buffets where you can pick up a ready-made lunch or dinner. It's also a great way to try new vegetables and flavors before committing to cooking up a whole batch at home.

Ultra-Easy Recipes

Some recipes are very quick. Try my hummus recipe, for example (page 127). In ten minutes, you'll have a batch that will make a week's worth of sandwiches. There are also recipes that are not really quick, but don't require *your* time. For the longest time I was reluctant to cook beans from scratch, figuring it took forever. But then I learned that they don't really need supervision (see "Cooking Beans" box). That goes for rice, too. My rice recipe is foolproof and delicious and requires more or less no hands-on effort (Perfect Brown Rice, page 136).

Cooking Beans

↠ **Yes, beans practically cook themselves. Starting with dry beans, soak them for at least 6 hours (or overnight), then discard the soaking water. Rinse the beans and add fresh water—at least twice as much water as beans. Bring to a boil and simmer until the beans are very soft, typically about 1½ hours. If you prefer, a pressure cooker will cook beans much more quickly, and an electric pressure cooker can be left unattended. You could also use a slow cooker. While they are cooking, you can do something else, and you will have plenty to divide up into serving-size bowls for later use.** ↞

Grocery and Meal Delivery Services

Many grocery stores are eager to deliver straight to your door. Just put in your order online, and the groceries arrive in the timeslot that you choose. You will also find meal delivery services that provide recipes with premeasured ingredients, ready to be whipped together when you are ready.

Cook on the Weekend

Make a big batch of soup, lasagna, or whatever else you fancy on Saturday or Sunday, and divide it into portions for the week ahead. You can even make enough to freeze portions so that you can grab and defrost a terrific homemade meal when you're short on time.

Tips for Shopping and Saving Money

Some people imagine that vegan foods are pricey. That might be true for organic hand-rolled asparagus sushi or any other exotic product, vegan or not. But as a rule of thumb, vegan foods are the cheapest ones in the store. Think about it. A bag of dried beans or rice costs pennies. A sack of sweet potatoes is cheap, as are those blocks of frozen vegetables and canned beans. Since you are skipping meat, cheese, and other nonvegan foods, you'll save plenty. Many stores have bulk aisles where you'll save even more.

Check the Food Label

While you're at the store, check the food label on any items that are new to you. If this seems time-consuming, take heart—you only need to check each product once, and some manufacturers make things easy by printing "vegan" right up front on the ingredients list.

The ingredients are listed by weight, starting with the ingredient used in the greatest amount. See if there are any animal products, such as milk, eggs, or their derivatives (casein, caseinate, whey, albumin, or lactalbumin).

The nutrition facts label lists cholesterol, which should be zero (cholesterol comes from animal products), and saturated fat, which should be close to zero. If weight loss is your goal, check the total fat number, too. You'll want to favor products with no more than 2 to 3 grams of fat per serving. By the way, if the listed serving size is, say, one cookie and you normally eat two cookies, double the amount of fat per serving for an accurate sense of what you'll actually be consuming. Sodium numbers vary widely from product to product. For

Nutrition Facts

Serving Size 1 cup (245g)
Servings Per Container About 2

Amount Per Serving	
Calories 90	Calories from Fat 0

	% Daily Value*
Total Fat 1.5g	**2%**
Saturated Fat 0g	**0%**
Trans Fat 0g	
Cholesterol 0mg	**0%**
Sodium 290mg	**12%**
Total Carbohydrate 17g	**6%**
Dietary Fiber 3g	**12%**
Sugars 5g	
Protein 3g	

Vitamin A 6%	•	Vitamin C 6%
Calcium 2%	•	Iron 6%

*Percent Daily Values are based on a 2,000 calorie diet.

context, most health authorities recommend limiting sodium to 1,500 to 2,000 milligrams per day.

Let's illustrate with a can of minestrone. The ingredients list starts with water, followed by diced tomatoes, diced onions, carrots, kidney beans, potatoes, and celery, and there are no animal products listed. The nutrition facts label (page 74) lists the cholesterol content as zero, as we'd expect. The saturated fat content is also zero (your heart is happy about that), and total fat is only 1.5 grams in a 1-cup serving, so that's good, too. The sodium content, 290 milligrams, is fine. So this product is indeed vegan, low in fat, and a good choice.

So, as you have seen, a vegan diet does not require spending any more time in the kitchen than you want to. It fits into any lifestyle. In the next chapter, we will have a look at healthy eating when you are on the road or out on the town.

CHAPTER 8

On the Go:
Work, Restaurants, Travel,
and Parties

MORE AND MORE OF OUR MEALS ARE EATEN OUTSIDE THE home—at work, at restaurants, or on the road. Let's look at how to find vegan choices wherever you are.

Healthy Food at Work

It is getting easier and easier to eat well at work. Most workplaces have a refrigerator and microwave, so heating up a frozen meal, a canned soup, or leftovers is a snap. If you don't have access to either of those things, it's still easy to stick to a healthy meal plan. Here are a few other things to keep on hand:

> ➤ **If your work environment doesn't give you easy access to a refrigerator or microwave, never fear! Insulated food storage containers keep your hot foods hot and cold foods cold for hours at a time.** ◀

Hummus. Make your own (page 127) or pick it up at the store and keep it in the refrigerator, ready to turn into a sandwich with lettuce and tomato or a dip with crackers.

Soups. Keep a package of soup in your desk drawer, and you'll always have an easy meal on hand. Whether from a can or a dry soup packet, almost any grocery store or food supplier will have plenty of choices to keep your meals varied and appealing.

Fresh fruit. Bananas, oranges, apples, pears, grapes, and raisins are healthful snacks that travel well. Keep extra on hand to share.

Sandwiches. Make a BLT with veggie bacon or tempeh, or a CLT, with cucumbers. Or pile on lettuce, tomato, and a vegan meat substitute, along with mustard or vegan mayo.

Rice bowl. At home, put cooked brown rice (see Perfect Brown Rice recipe on page 136) in a sealable microwavable bowl and add cooked broccoli or other green vegetables, plus almonds, chickpeas, tofu, or other toppings, drizzled with soy sauce. You can even prepare these foods in batches and divide them into containers so that you can grab a tasty prepared meal from your refrigerator throughout the week.

Parties at Work

When your office is celebrating, bring some vegan ice cream, fresh fruit, baked chips and salsa, or something else to share. If the office celebration is at a restaurant, talk to the planning committee about restaurant choices, and consider calling the restaurant ahead of time to make sure that they have what you are looking for.

Company Cafeteria

Company cafeterias can easily serve vegan choices: an oatmeal bar for breakfast and a salad bar for lunch, vegetable or split pea soup, vegan chili, veggie burgers, and plenty of vegetables and fresh fruit. If your cafeteria does not have good choices, let the cafeteria manager know that you and your coworkers are eager for an expanded menu and will make it pay off.

Healthy Food at Restaurants

There are more and more great vegan restaurants nowadays. Fort Lauderdale's famed Sublime set the standard, under the watchful eye of owner Nanci Alexander, with waterfalls, original paintings, and a diverse vegan menu from top to bottom. Now many others have followed suit. All over the world, diners are now finding vegan restaurants, from casual to elegant, in their neighborhoods. When it comes to not-yet-vegan restaurants, nearly all serve vegan meals, and chefs are getting more and more creative all the time. Here are some ideas:

Italian restaurants feature endless vegan choices, starting with bruschetta and delicious salads and soups (minestrone, lentil, and pasta e fagioli), followed by spaghetti, angel hair, or other pastas topped with sautéed mushrooms, artichoke hearts, and arrabbiata or marinara sauce, along with grilled asparagus, spinach, or other healthful vegetables. Just ask the server to leave off the cheese and steer clear of cream-based sauces.

➤ You may need to ask chefs to restrain their exuberance for olive oil. They sometimes go way too far with it, a trait common to many cuisines. ➤

Pizza restaurants are used to diners asking for no cheese and extra tomato sauce, plus mushrooms, spinach, olives, onions, bell peppers, and jalapeños. If you're sharing a pizza with someone who isn't willing to try it your way, you can ask for the cheese, meat, or other nonvegan ingredients on just half the pie and get the other half how you like it.

Chinese restaurants (including Hunan, Szechuan, and Cantonese) feature delicious dishes made from vegetables, tofu, rice, and noodles and sometimes offer "mock meats." Some even have special menus normally offered to Chinese diners, featuring a wide range of savory green vegetables sautéed with garlic. Have plenty of rice and use the main dish as a flavorful topping.

Mexican restaurants serve bean burritos, veggie fajitas, spinach enchiladas, and beans and rice with spicy salsa and often have fresh tropical fruits. If the restaurant still uses lard in their beans, on the theory that it is somehow a "traditional" flavoring, you might remind them that Native Americans were cooking beans in the Americas long before the Spanish brought pigs and cholesterol with them.

Japanese restaurants are especially good choices. Not only do they feature many plant-based foods, all delicately flavored; they also use very little oil. Start with edamame and a green salad or seaweed salad, followed by sushi rolls made of cucumber, asparagus, tofu, or other plant-based ingredients. Miso soup is often vegan, although not always, so you will want to ask.

Vietnamese, Thai, and other Asian restaurants offer delicate dishes made from rice, vegetables, tofu, and delicious sauces. You'll find savory soups, spring rolls, crepes, garlic-sautéed vegetables, and plenty of noodle dishes. They will gladly omit the animal ingredients for you.

Middle Eastern restaurants feature falafel, hummus, tabbouleh, and couscous, along with many other tasty choices. With plenty of spices, herbs, and flavorful preparations, this is a great cuisine to try if you're looking for something filling and delicious.

Indian restaurants always feature vegetarian cuisine: samosas, popadams, dal, and main dishes made from spinach, lentils, chickpeas, potatoes, and other healthful vegetables. Their main weak point is a tendency to drench foods in milk, ghee, or oil, none of which will do your arteries or waistline any good. Happily, many are now preparing vegan dishes that are much lower in oil, and most will prepare any dish without milk or ghee upon request.

Ethiopian restaurants feature simple, savory dishes made from lentils, split peas, potatoes, green beans, cabbage, tomatoes, and hot peppers served on injera, a soft flatbread.

Steak houses may be where your friends or family convene. Perhaps surprisingly, steak houses often take pride in their vegetables, and their managers are well aware that some diners are looking for vegan choices. Ask for a vegetable plate, a baked potato with salsa or marinara sauce, or a pasta dish.

Fast Foods

Many fast-food restaurants offer vegan options, which are often the cheapest items on the menu. Here are a few:

Taco restaurants offer bean burritos and veggie burritos and will gladly substitute beans for meat on tacos. Skip the cheese and add sliced jalapeños, lettuce, tomatoes, onions, or whatever else you like. There are lots of other ways to veganize their offerings. For example, starting with Taco Bell's 7-Layer Burrito, just skip the cheese and sour cream. Chipotle will gladly build a thoroughly stuffed vegan taco or black bean burrito.

Sandwich shops, like Subway and Quiznos, usually have a whole bar of vegetables to choose from and will stuff a sandwich with lettuce, tomato, cucumbers, olives, spinach, peppers, and maybe sautéed mushrooms. Sprinkle red wine vinegar over the top for extra flavor. They will even toast it for you.

Burger restaurants often serve veggie burgers. Wendy's offers baked potatoes, which you can top with steamed vegetables.

Family-style restaurants, like Denny's or Bob Evans, offer veggie burgers, pasta dishes, and plenty of side vegetables that can be combined to make a vegetable plate.

Salad bars. Grocery stores are not fast-food restaurants, but many have food that is really fast. Check out their salad bars featuring hot and cold offerings. You can pick up a meal and be on your way in minutes.

Restaurant Tricks

The diner breakfast. Yes, diners serve oatmeal and grits. But how about asking for mushrooms, spinach, asparagus, tomatoes, or onions on the grill—all the things that would normally go in an omelet, minus the omelet—along with rye toast (hold the butter) and breakfast potatoes?

Healthful dressings. Typical salad dressings and sauces are fatty and loaded with calories, and some contain animal products like cheese or bacon. Better choices include balsamic vinegar, seasoned rice vinegar, or lemon juice squeezed from fresh wedges. And if you ask that dressings and sauces be served on the side, you'll be able to control how much goes on. Sprinkle on as much pepper as you like for a little extra heat.

❖

➤ Most restaurants can easily accommodate vegan requests, and "international" restaurants of all stripes make vegan eating really easy no matter where you are. But if you want to dig in a bit more, the Internet is your friend. You can check restaurant menus online (although sometimes the web versions show only a portion of the restaurant's capabilities). When you're headed to a new city, you might do a Google or Yelp search for vegan restaurants in the area. There are also websites and apps (e.g., HappyCow, VeganXpress, Vegan NYC) to help you. Since restaurants are opening and closing day by day, it pays to call before you go. ◀

❖

➤ Be sure to tip generously at restaurants. Your bill is likely the smallest one your server will have all day, so a typical percentage tip might be a little light, especially if your server has gone the extra mile for you. Your generosity will give vegans a good name. ◀

Travel

The key to healthy eating on the road is to plan ahead. Here are a few tips:

In your car. You can, of course, stop at fast-food places along the way—using the list in the previous section. You might also want to bring food in your car:

- ☞ Bananas, apples, or other car-friendly fruit
- ☞ Luna Bars, low-fat granola bars, or trail mix
- ☞ Dried fruit
- ☞ Applesauce or fruit cups
- ☞ Baby carrots and sliced cucumbers
- ☞ Rice cakes and bean dip
- ☞ Small soy milk or almond milk cartons
- ☞ PB & J sandwiches

In the air. Overseas flights offer vegan meals, provided you call at least forty-eight hours before flight time. On domestic flights, snack service is limited—you might find hummus and crackers, for example—so you're better off packing a sandwich or picking up some bananas at the airport.

At your hotel. Midpriced hotels in the United States typically have in-room refrigerators and microwaves (ask when you reserve). That way, you can drop by a nearby grocery store and stock up on frozen dinners, fresh fruit, instant soups, canned beans, or whatever your taste calls for, or save leftovers from a restaurant meal. For extra credit, pick up a good-size bowl and a small box of oatmeal at the grocery store, and you're set for the morning. Some extended-stay hotels have full kitchens.

> ➤ When you order at a restaurant or from room service, remember that the menu is just a suggestion. The cook can usually whip up oatmeal or throw some asparagus, mushrooms, and tomatoes on the grill for breakfast, even if they are not listed. They probably can do spaghetti with tomato sauce, a vegetable plate, or veggie burgers for lunch or dinner. Don't be afraid to ask and you'll be pleasantly surprised by what you find. ➤

Partying Without Missing a Beat

Let's say you're invited to a party, and you're wondering what kind of challenge this might pose to your healthful-eating resolve. Will there be anything to eat? Will you refuse the unhealthy offerings and hurt your host's feelings? Not to worry. Here are a few tips that will make it a breeze:

Offer to bring something. The worst thing is to not tell your hosts about your vegan diet; if they find out later, they will feel that they have been bad hosts. If you receive an invitation to a dinner party, let your hosts know in advance that you are following a vegan diet and that you don't want to be a bother. Then ask if you can bring a food gift. Of course, your hosts will say no, there will be plenty to eat. But now you've let them know in the politest possible way about your eating preferences.

Bring a gift. Arriving at a party with a gift of fruit, a selection of dips, a loaf of special bread, or some other food gift is a polite gesture. And if your hosts open it up, they've just enlarged the vegan options for the party.

Don't arrive ravenous. You are going to a party to see friends or family, not to stuff yourself. So if you are famished, have a snack before you go so that you're not dependent on someone else's menu.

When your host is a little too pushy. Once in a while a host can be a little overbearing, pushing you to eat something you'd rather skip. Keep in mind, hosts don't really care if you eat or not; they just want to be good hosts. So keep a plate in your hand with something on it (hosts like to fill empty plates), and pay them an honest compliment or two to take the focus off you.

Are Others Feeling Guilty?

When others find out you are not eating animal products, they may feel self-conscious or even a little guilty. They might launch into an unsolicited soliloquy that starts with "I'd say I only eat meat maybe twice a month…" They might be argumentative: "Do you wear leather shoes?" "Aren't humans supposed to eat meat?" Not that you asked for any of this. They just want to spill out their thoughts.

My suggestion is to briefly offer your experience if you like and mention a book, such as this one, or a movie or website that you have found helpful, and then leave it at that. Do feel free to share, but don't proselytize. Once you've planted a seed, it will germinate in its own time.

This is another nice reason why gifts are good. When you bring a gift for others to try, you'll melt through any doubts and keep things positive.

CHAPTER 9

Bumps in the Road

A VEGAN DIET BRINGS ABUNDANT REWARDS AND MOST PEOPLE find it much easier than they imagined. Even so, setting off on a new path can bring an occasional bump in the road. Let's tackle the unexpected issues that can come up.

I'm Not Losing Weight Fast Enough

A vegan diet usually helps people lose unwanted weight more or less automatically. But if that's not happening—or it's not happening fast enough—here are a few things to check:

1. Be sure you are avoiding animal products *completely*. Even small amounts of meat or cheese can stymie your weight loss. Remember, they have fat and calories with no appetite-taming fiber at all.

2. Do a search-and-destroy mission for oily foods. Remember, every gram of fat or oil holds 9 calories, and that goes even for "good" fats. So if oils, nuts, or avocados figure big in your life, your weight is likely to get stuck.

3. Do not avoid healthful carbohydrates. Some people are afraid of rice or sweet potatoes, imagining them to be fattening. But

keep in mind, these foods kept Asians slim for centuries, until Western dietary habits escorted meat, milk, and cheese into these countries. Where people sometimes run into trouble is with fatty toppings—butter on bread, gravy on rice, and so forth. So be mindful of how you're serving them, but don't avoid healthful carbohydrates.

4. Have more raw food. Fresh fruit, carrots, and salads are naturally filling and low in calories.

5. Make sure you are well hydrated. Sometimes thirst is misinterpreted as hunger.

6. Have soup! Most vegan soups (except creamy varieties) are naturally modest in calories and very filling.

7. Avoid late-evening eating. Go to bed.

8. Don't count on exercise for weight loss. Exercise has many benefits, but its weight-loss effect is modest. It does not take the place of changing what's on your plate.

I'm Losing Too Much Weight

If you feel you are becoming too thin, you might first check your body mass index (BMI) to see if your weight is in the healthy range or not. You can do this easily with any online BMI calculator. If the result is between 18.5 and 24.9, you are in the healthy range.

If you really are underweight, check with your health care provider to see if there is a medical issue to address. If it is just a question of inadequate calories, start with larger servings of healthful grains, vegetables, beans, and fruit. You might also want to consider weight-bearing exercise to help preserve your muscle mass.

If you are determined to gain weight, adding nuts and other fatty foods to your diet is likely to bring on some weight, although it might end up around your midsection, rather than where you want it.

My Family and Friends Don't Support Me

This can happen, and solving it is important, not just for you, but for them, too. Families and friends often take their cues from one another about what is healthy and what is not. So, for example, if one spouse gains weight, the other may as well.[22] But it works the other way, too: If you set off on a healthier path, your family and friends may well follow.

Sometimes, you do have to remind your friends why you are improving your eating habits. One of our research participants taught me a great trick. One of her coworkers had been making fun of her vegan diet and was tempting her with all manner of foods that she did not want to eat. Here's how she handled it: She sat her coworker down and said words to this effect, "You've always been there for me, and I want to ask your help with something really important to me. I'm switching to a vegan diet for my health. And I'm afraid I'll be tempted by things, or that other people might forget and might tempt me with foods I'm trying to stay away from. So if you see someone doing that, could you maybe have a quiet word with them?" It worked like a charm. Her coworker became her defender and ally.

The best thing, of course, is for your family and friends to join you for, say, a three-week "test drive" of a vegan diet. Invite them to do it, and keep the focus on the short term, so the experiment stays approachable and fun.

If you are the cook in the family, I would encourage you not to feel any need to make two meals for your family—a vegan one for you and meat for them. If the meals you serve are tasty, everyone can eat healthful vegan foods. That is especially true for children. Even if a healthy diet is a bit new to you and to them, it pays to approach it with the same confidence that you would have about not allowing smoking or drug use in your home.

If you need more support, you might wish to enlarge your network by joining online communities, attending a local cooking class or vegetarian event, or treating yourself to a vegan cruise, where you will meet hundreds of like-minded people.

I Need More Options

If you are feeling like your range of foods has narrowed, it is time to branch out. Look at international restaurants serving Italian, Mexican, Chinese, Japanese, Thai, and the other cuisines we've talked about. There is a similar array in the freezer case at natural food stores and regular groceries and in the recipes you'll find online and in cookbooks.

My Blood Sugar or Triglycerides Went Up

If you have type 2 diabetes, it is likely to improve dramatically and may even disappear when you get the animal products and added oils out of your diet. However, for the first few days on a vegan diet, your blood sugars could be higher than before. As we saw in Chapter 4, this is because fat inside your muscle and liver cells has made them *insulin-resistant*, so just about any starchy or sweet food will raise your blood sugar. If you stick with a low-fat vegan diet, this will soon pass, and you should see your numbers improving. As I mentioned earlier, be sure to let your caregiver know that you are improving your diet; before long, your need for medication may change.

Triglycerides can sometimes rise, too. If that happens for you, you will want to take care to avoid all animal products and added fats, and also to avoid added sugars and high-Glycemic-Index foods (see Chapter 4).

I Really Crave Cheese, Meat, or Junk Food

This, too, will pass. Focus on the short term and avoid them completely. Having the occasional nonvegan indulgence will only reawaken your cravings. If you really feel like you need something, vegan substitutes (vegan cheese, veggie bacon, etc.) are okay. But be choosy. Food manufacturers have found ways to make vegan versions of all the things that are fattening your not-yet-vegan friends: ice creams, cakes, cookies, sausages, and so on. These vegan treats are not necessarily forbidden, but read the labels, and, as a general rule, you will want to favor simple, healthful foods.

My Doctor (or Other Caregiver) Does Not Understand a Vegan Diet

Unfortunately, many doctors grew up with less-than-healthy eating habits, just like everyone else, and nutrition is neglected in medical education. If your caregiver is not knowledgeable or not sympathetic to a vegan diet, you can share this book with him or her. And there is an abundance of nutrition materials at the Physicians Committee for Responsible Medicine's website (pcrm.org), including scientific reports, continuing medical education, and conference information.

I'm Gassy

First, be sure you have scrapped dairy products completely; milk sugar (lactose) can cause gassiness and diarrhea. Among plant-based foods, the main culprits are beans and undercooked cruciferous vegetables (e.g., broccoli, cauliflower, cabbage, and Brussels sprouts). Have smaller servings, and be sure they are well cooked. If you are cooking beans from scratch, it helps to discard the soaking water and to cook them thoroughly. Over time, as your digestive bacteria get healthier, you'll likely find that your digestion sorts itself out.

Also, steer clear of fatty foods (e.g., potato chips) and sugary foods, as they can affect your digestive health, too. Have more brown rice, pasta, and simple starchy vegetables.

I Need More Energy

If you are feeling a little low on energy, try these tips:

First, be sure you are getting enough sleep. Turn out the lights at 10 p.m. instead of staying up late.

Second, be sure to eat *enough*. If you are not eating adequate portions, you can run out of fuel before your next meal.

Third, have higher-protein foods early in the day and early at each meal. Beans, tofu, or meat substitutes provide plenty of healthful protein that can help you stay alert. Here is why: High-carbohydrate foods can cause the brain to produce *serotonin*, a natural brain chemical that causes calmness and sometimes sleepiness. Protein—in beans, tofu, tempeh, soy milk, or other higher-protein foods—blocks this effect. You can do the opposite when you want to sleep: Have white bread or another starchy food. Your brain will make a bit of serotonin to help you doze off.

Fourth, ditch caffeine. Caffeine is a stimulant, of course. But many people become habituated to it, finding that they have less energy overall than they did before caffeine entered their lives. Picture children: They have boundless energy and don't need a shot of espresso to pick up their energy. Because they are never in caffeine withdrawal, they have more energy.

Can Dogs and Cats Be Vegan?

Yes. A vegan diet is possible and even advantageous, particularly considering what ends up in meat-based commercial dog food and cat food brands. Most dogs go vegan relatively easily and thrive. Cats are more finicky and have more challenging nutritional needs, requiring taurine and vitamin A supplements. I would encourage you to buy food products and supplements specifically designed for vegan dogs and cats. Several companies sell them, and you will find more details at the website for People for the Ethical Treatment of Animals (peta.org).

CHAPTER 10

Favorite Myths

THERE IS A WEALTH OF SCIENTIFIC SUPPORT FOR PLANT-BASED diets, so much so that the American Medical Association has called for vegan meals to be served in schools, hospitals, and food assistance programs, and the US government and the Academy of Nutrition and Dietetics stand behind their health power. Even so, lots of nutrition myths linger. This chapter tackles them.

Myth #1: It's Hard to Go Vegan

A vegan diet does require learning a few new tricks. But most people find it much easier than low-calorie diets that leave you hungry most of the time, or low-carb diets that ban bread, potatoes, spaghetti, fruit, beans, and so many other foods that you are left feeling unsatisfied. Breaking a meat and dairy habit is *much* easier than quitting smoking or breaking other bad habits. Often, it's just a matter of modifying the foods you are eating now. Very soon, it will feel more or less effortless. And because, over time, you'll find yourself exploring new tastes and new cuisines from around the world, your range of foods seems larger, not smaller.

Myth #2: Carbohydrates Are Fattening

There is a reason that people on traditional Asian diets are slim: The rice, noodles, and starchy vegetables that are their staples are naturally low in calories. As you now know, carbohydrates have only 4 calories per gram, compared with 9 for fats and oils. Sometimes, when people blame carbs for weight gain that comes from eating cakes and cookies, the real culprit is the butter or shortening hiding inside, which is much more fattening than the flour or sugar.

Myth #3: You Can't Get Enough Protein on a Vegan Diet

This myth just will not die, despite (1) statements supporting vegan diets from major nutrition organizations, (2) the wealth of protein in beans, vegetables, and grains, (3) the massive musculature of rhinoceroses, elephants, and other vegan animals, and (4) the millions of people following vegan diets with no evidence that protein is an issue at all. If this myth is still reverberating in your mind, have another look at Chapter 5.

Myth #4: Soy Causes Cancer

Decades ago, scientists found natural compounds, called *isoflavones*, in soybeans and many other foods. Because their chemical structure vaguely resembles the sex hormones estrogen and testosterone, some people have called these compounds "phytoestrogens"—meaning "plant estrogens"—raising the question as to whether soy products might cause breast cancer. I discussed this in Chapter 4, but since the myth lives on, let's tackle it in more depth.

Researchers have tracked the diets of thousands of women, observing that women consuming the most soy (soy milk, tofu, etc.) are *less* likely to develop breast cancer, compared with those having the least soy in their diets. The protective effect is on the order of 30 to 40 percent.[10,11] It also turns out that, among women who have been previously treated for breast cancer, soy products reduce the risk of cancer recurrence.[12]

Soy products are not essential, but they are handy. Far from causing cancer, they help prevent cancer and reduce the risk of recurrence in women who have had cancer previously.

Myth #5: You Should Base Your Diet on Your Blood Type

In 1996, the book *Eat Right for Your Type* suggested that people with type A blood should be vegetarian, while people with type O blood needed meat, and there were other diet suggestions for blood types B and AB. That notion quickly ran aground. First, type O is the most common blood type. And in research studies, type O people improve their health on the vegan diet, just as type A people do. Meat does not make them healthier.

So I am writing a new book, called *Eat Right for Your Shoe Size*, suggesting that if you wear a 9½, you would do well on a vegan diet. If you take a 10 or 11, you would do well on a vegan diet, too.

Myth #6: All Foods Can Be Eaten "in Moderation"

This risky myth keeps unhealthy foods on many people's plates. But studies show that people eating modest amounts of animal products are heavier, have a higher risk of diabetes, and have much more trouble reversing their health problems, compared with people who skip these products altogether.

"Moderation" should apply only to healthful things. If your daughter loves to play the violin, you would certainly encourage her. But after six or eight hours of practice, she needs to eat dinner, do her homework, or have a bit of exercise. Playing the violin is great, but it needs to be done in moderation. If your son loves broccoli, he should not eat *only* broccoli. He needs other healthful foods, too. So moderation makes sense here, too.

But how many cigarettes should your kids smoke? How much cocaine should they have? Moderation applies to *healthful* things, not to dangerous things.

Myth #7: Children Might Not Get Adequate Nutrition on a Vegan Diet

As we saw in Chapter 6, children raised on plant-based diets have *better diets and better health*, compared with children whose diets include meat, cheese, and other nonvegan foods. And the rules are simple: Build the menu from our healthy staples—vegetables, fruits, whole grains, and legumes—and be sure to include a vitamin B_{12} supplement. Hopefully your children are getting out into the sunlight more or less every day. If not, they will also need vitamin D. That's about it. For details, have another look at Chapter 6.

Myth #8: Vegan Food Is Expensive

If you subscribe to this notion, pop into the nearest sandwich shop and ask the price of a sandwich without meat and cheese. It's cheaper than everything else. Now head for the nearest taco shop and see what a bean burrito costs, compared with a chicken or beef version. Not a penny more—and maybe less. Now drop in at the grocery store and check out the price of dried beans, rice, canned and frozen vegetables, sweet potatoes, and other simple foods. As you will see, everything is pretty cheap.

What gets expensive is preparation. If you are paying for someone else to turn an avocado and bread into a sandwich at the store, it will cost more than the ingredients alone, just as it would for tuna or beef. In other words, it is not the vegan food that was pricey; it was the preparation time. Overall, studies show that plant-based eating is substantially cheaper than diets that include animal products. And if you've been able to reduce your need for medications or other treatments, you're saving serious money. This book has some time-saving tips, such as batch cooking and fast recipes; if you need more, you'll be amazed at how many tips you'll find online with some quick searching.

Myth #9: Athletes Need Meat

We touched on this briefly in Chapter 4. Endurance athletes get an energy boost when they set aside the animal products, because their tissues oxygenate better when there is no animal fat to slow blood flow.

If you think that animal protein somehow builds better muscle than plant protein, have a look at Patrik Baboumian. Often called the world's strongest man, he set a world record in 2015 by lifting 1,232 pounds and carrying it for twenty-eight seconds (don't try this at home). He got his enormous musculature the way bulls and elephants get theirs—entirely from plants. Eating muscles does not give you muscles any more than eating brains makes you smart. Athletes need some protein—and plants deliver plenty of complete protein. A gazelle would not run faster if it ate bacon, and an elephant would not have greater strength or bigger muscles if it ate an omelet, steak, or fried chicken.

Myth #10: Humans Are Natural Carnivores

The Paleo diet craze provides the romantic image that our loincloth-clad forebears were skilled hunters, ready for the cover of *Men's Health*. The biological truth is that we are great apes, in the same category as gorillas, orangutans, chimpanzees, and bonobos, all of whom build their diets either largely or entirely from plant sources.

True carnivores—like cheetahs and lions—are quick on their feet and able to catch prey and dismember it with sharp claws and canine teeth. But we are not particularly fast and have no claws, and our canine teeth are no longer than our incisors. But when the Stone Age arrived, everything changed. We were able to fashion arrow-heads and spears that were faster than we were, and we were able to make stone tools that could kill and tear apart prey. The problem is that we have pre–Stone Age coronary arteries and intestinal tracts, and meat causes problems for us that it does not cause for dogs, cats, and other true carnivores.

Acknowledgments

THANK YOU TO THE THOUSANDS OF PARTICIPANTS IN RESEARCH studies and to the staff of the Physicians Committee for Responsible Medicine who helped establish the health power of vegan diets. Thanks to Susan Levin, MS, RD, for her guidance on complete nutrition for children. The recipes come through the generosity of Christine Waltermyer; Hana Kahleova, MD, PhD; Dora Stone; Rose Saltalamacchia; Lee Crosby, RD; Noah Kauffman; Karen Smith, RD; Caroline Trapp, DNP; Maggie Neola, RD; and Naif Hérin, and Christine tested them all carefully. I am very grateful to all of you! Thanks also to Jill Eckart, CHC; Susan Levin, MS, RD; Lee Crosby, RD; Andrea Cimino; Hana Kahleova, MD, PhD; Karen Smith, RD; Maggie Neola, RD; Noah Kauffman; Erica Nielson; Ashley Waddell; Sonia Hawkins; and Laura Anderson for reviewing the text. Thank you to Amber Green, RD, for handling all the nutrient analyses. Thank you to my literary agent, Brian DeFiore, and my editor, Leah Miller, for their expertise and wonderful support of this book.

Recommended Resources

Let me recommend some books, cookbooks, and websites for further reading. When it comes to my own titles, here are a few that focus on special topics and may be helpful to you:

21-Day Weight Loss Kickstart (New York: Grand Central Publishing, 2011).

Dr. Neal Barnard's Program for Reversing Diabetes (Emmaus, PA: Rodale, 2018).

Foods That Fight Pain (New York: Harmony/Random House, 1998).

Power Foods for the Brain (New York: Grand Central Publishing, 2013).

The Cancer Survivor's Guide, co-authored with Jennifer K. Reilly (Summertown, TN: Healthy Living Publications, 2008).

The Cheese Trap (New York: Grand Central Publishing, 2017).

And here are two cookbooks:

Dr. Neal Barnard's Cookbook for Reversing Diabetes (Emmaus, PA: Rodale, 2018).

The Get Healthy, Go Vegan Cookbook, co-authored with Robyn Webb (Boston: Da Capo, 2010).

There are great books by other authors as well—more than I can list here. But here are several that have inspired and informed many people:

Health and Nutrition Books

T. Colin Campbell and Thomas M. Campbell II, *The China Study* (Dallas, TX: BenBella Books, 2006).

Brenda Davis and Vesanto Melina, *Becoming Vegan* (Summertown, TN: Book Publishing Company, 2014).

Caldwell Esselstyn, *Prevent and Reverse Heart Disease* (New York: Avery, 2007).

Rip Esselstyn, *The Engine 2 Diet* (New York: Grand Central Publishing, 2009).

Kathy Freston and Bruce Friedrich, *Clean Protein* (New York: Hachette, 2018).

Michael Greger, *How Not to Die* (New York: Flatiron Books, 2015).

Micaela Cook Karlsen, *A Plant-Based Life* (New York: AMACOM, 2016).

Reed Mangels, *The Everything Vegan Pregnancy Book* (Avon, MA: Adams Media, 2011).

John A. McDougall and Mary McDougall, *The Starch Solution* (Emmaus, PA: Rodale, 2012).

Victoria Moran and Adair Moran, *Main Street Vegan* (New York: TarcherPerigee, 2012).

Lani Muelrath, *The Mindful Vegan* (Dallas, TX: BenBella Books, 2017).

Dean Ornish, *Dr. Dean Ornish's Program for Reversing Heart Disease* (New York: Ivy Books, 1995).

Alona Pulde and Matthew Lederman, *Forks Over Knives Family* (New York: Touchstone, 2016).

Will Tuttle, *The World Peace Diet* (Brooklyn, NY: Lantern Books, 2016).

Cookbooks

Dreena Burton, *Plant-Powered Families* (Dallas, TX: BenBella Books, 2015).

Rip Esselstyn and Jane Esselstyn, *The Engine 2 Cookbook* (New York: Grand Central Publishing, 2017).

Cathy Fisher, *Straight Up Food* (Santa Rosa, CA: Green Bite Publishing, 2016).

Michael Greger, *The How Not to Die Cookbook* (New York: Flatiron Books, 2017).

Richa Hingle, *Vegan Richa's Everyday Kitchen* (Woodstock, VA: Vegan Heritage Press, 2017).

Angela Liddon, *The Oh She Glows Cookbook* (New York: Avery, 2014).

Isa Chandra Moskowitz, *Isa Does It* (New York: Little, Brown and Company, 2013).

Lindsay Nixon, *The Happy Herbivore Cookbook* (Dallas, TX: BenBella Books, 2011).

Colleen Patrick-Goudreau, *The Vegan Table* (Beverly, MA: Fair Winds Press, 2009).

Rich Roll and Julie Piatt, *The Plantpower Way* (New York: Avery, 2015).

Del Sroufe, *Forks Over Knives—The Cookbook* (New York: Experiment, 2012).

Christine Waltermyer, *The Natural Vegan Kitchen* (Summertown, TN: Book Publishing Company, 2011).

Jason Wyrick, *Vegan Mexico* (Woodstock, VA: Vegan Heritage Press, 2016).

Websites

Physicians Committee for Responsible Medicine (pcrm.org) features a 21-Day Vegan Kickstart program, abundant nutrition information, and a great many free recipes.

Colleen Patrick-Goudreau (colleenpatrickgoudreau.com) has a popular podcast and many practical resources.

Fatfree Vegan Recipes (fatfreevegan.com) is just what it sounds like.

Finding Vegan (findingvegan.com), established by Kathy Patalsky, is a quick and fun way to find recipes from your favorite bloggers all in one place.

Forks Over Knives (forksoverknives.com) has great recipes, meal-planning tools, success stories, and more.

Isa Chandra (isachandra.com), created by Isa Chandra Moskowitz, has a super-practical ingredient-based recipe finder.

Lighter (lighter.world) shows you which foods to buy and how to throw great meals together, based on the recommendations of food leaders.

NutritionFacts.org brings you Dr. Michael Greger's vast nutrition knowledge in clever, easy-to-understand videos.

Oh She Glows (ohsheglows.com) is a practical recipe blog created by Angela Liddon.

Our Hen House (ourhenhouse.org) has inspiring podcasts with an ethical focus.

People for the Ethical Treatment of Animals (peta.org) has great information on vegan diets for companion animals, motivating information on ethical food choices, and tips on going vegan.

Pinterest (pinterest.com) lets you search for and save vegan recipes and offers you new ones the next time you visit.

Plant-Based on a Budget (plantbasedonabudget.com) shows how to make healthy eating economical.

Rich Roll (richroll.com) has an enormously popular podcast and plenty of inspiration and information.

The Vegan Corner (thevegancorner.com) is a source of unique oil-free vegan dishes presented with a sense of humor.

Vegan Richa (veganricha.com) is a great recipe resource from Richa Hingle.

Vegetarian Resource Group (vrg.org) has expert writers and great information for going vegan throughout the life cycle.

VegNews (vegnews.com) is *the* source for the latest in vegan culture, including great recipes.

Foods and Ingredients That May Be New to You

HUMMUS. Born in the Middle East, this spread made of chickpeas, tahini (ground sesame seeds), garlic, and various flavorings is a traditional breakfast food that also serves as a sandwich filling or dip. Grocery stores stock it, and you'll find a quick and easy recipe on page 127.

NUTRITIONAL YEAST. Found in the supplement or bulk aisle of natural food stores, nutritional yeast is bright yellow and adds a cheese-like flavor to pizza, pasta sauces, vegetables, and other foods.

SEITAN. Seitan (pronounced *SAY-tan*) is wheat protein (gluten) with a meaty texture. It is an ingredient in some veggie burgers and other products and is also sold in meaty shapes, ready to be added to stir-fries or other dishes.

SOY SAUCE and **TAMARI.** Both go great on rice, vegetables, and other dishes. So what's the difference? Soy sauce typically contains wheat. Tamari contains little or no wheat and may have a richer flavor. Reduced-sodium brands are widely available.

TEMPEH. Tempeh (pronounced *TEM-pay*) is a block of fermented soybeans. Like tofu, it readily takes up sauces and marinades and adds a meaty texture to dishes. You will find it in natural food stores and Asian markets.

TOFU. Very similar to cooked egg white, tofu does not have much taste on its own. But cooks love it for recipes where a little extra protein helps—like sauces and puddings. At breakfast, grilled or scrambled tofu is a healthy substitute for scrambled eggs, and Asian restaurants transform it into endless delectable traditional dishes. It is sold at all grocery stores. Firm tofu is often grilled or used in soups and stir-fries. Silken tofu lends itself to puddings and other soft-textured foods.

Recipes

Bircher Muesli

MAKES 4 SERVINGS

2 cups rolled oats

2 apples, grated

2 cups plain nondairy yogurt

3 tablespoons raisins

1 teaspoon ground cinnamon

Maple syrup, chia seeds, vanilla (optional)

Combine the oats, apples, yogurt, raisins, and cinnamon in a bowl. Cover and place in the refrigerator overnight. In the morning, divide into 4 bowls and serve with a drizzle of maple syrup or other optional toppings, if desired.

Per serving (¼ of recipe): 309 calories, 9 g protein, 59 g carbohydrate, 21 g sugar, 5 g fat, 14% calories from fat, 7 g fiber, 29 mg sodium

Recipe by Hana Kahleova

Carrot Cake Muffins

MAKES 12 SERVINGS

2 tablespoons ground flaxseed

5 tablespoons water

¾ cup almond milk or other nondairy milk

¾ cup unsweetened applesauce

½ cup maple syrup

1 teaspoon vanilla extract

1½ cups whole wheat flour

½ cup rolled oats

1 teaspoon baking soda

1½ teaspoons baking powder

Pinch of sea salt

1 teaspoon ground cinnamon

¼ teaspoon ground ginger

1 cup grated carrot

Vegetable oil spray

Preheat the oven to 350°F. Place the ground flaxseed in a small bowl and pour the water over it. Mix with a fork to incorporate and let stand for 5 minutes. Add the almond milk, applesauce, maple syrup, and vanilla extract to the bowl with the flaxseed mixture, and mix well. In a large bowl, combine the flour, oats, baking soda, baking powder, salt, cinnamon, and ginger. Mix well. Pour the flaxseed mixture into the large bowl with the flour. Mix until incorporated. Add the grated carrot. Mix to incorporate.

Lightly spray a muffin tin with vegetable oil spray or use muffin liners. Evenly divide the muffin batter into the muffin molds by filling up to three-quarters capacity. An ice cream scoop works well for this. Bake for 25 minutes or until a toothpick inserted into the muffin comes out clean.

Per serving (¹⁄₁₂ of recipe): 121 calories, 3 g protein, 26 g carbohydrate, 10 g sugar, 1 g fat, 10% calories from fat, 3 g fiber, 209 mg sodium

Recipe by Dora Stone

Easy Tofu Scramble

MAKES 2 SERVINGS

1 (14-ounce) block extra-firm tofu

1 tablespoon vegetable broth or soy sauce

½ green bell pepper, chopped

½ red bell pepper, chopped

½ medium onion, chopped

⅛ teaspoon sea salt

Black pepper, to taste

½ teaspoon turmeric, or 1 to 2 teaspoons curry powder,
       or to taste

Rinse the tofu and drain any excess water so that the tofu is as dry as possible. Break the tofu block into pieces with a fork to create a "scrambled" texture.

Heat a large frying pan over medium heat. Add the vegetable broth, bell peppers, onion, and salt. Cook and stir for 5 minutes, until the vegetables have softened slightly. Add the tofu, black pepper, and turmeric. Cook uncovered for another 10 to 15 minutes, or until slightly brown. Stir often while cooking. The longer the cooking time, the drier the scramble will be.

Note: Also try mushrooms or other vegetables in this dish.

Per serving (½ of recipe): 194 calories, 21 g protein, 9 g carbohydrate, 5 g sugar, 11 g fat, 46% calories from fat, 2 g fiber, 178 mg sodium

Recipe by Hana Kahleova

Breakfast Grillers

MAKES 4 SERVINGS

8 ounces uncooked tempeh

2 tablespoons low-sodium tamari or soy sauce

1 teaspoon liquid smoke

Cut the tempeh into strips, as follows: If you are using a typical 3 x 7-inch tempeh block, cut it crosswise into quarters, then turn each quarter into two thin strips by carefully slicing it down the middle, the thin way. In a small bowl, combine the tamari and liquid smoke. Place the tempeh strips on a plate and brush each strip with the tamari or soy sauce mixture. Let stand for 1 minute. Then, lay the strips in a hot frying pan (typically no oil is needed, but a light coating of cooking spray can be used if desired). Cook on medium-high heat until brown on one side (about 5 minutes), then turn to brown on the other side (another 5 minutes). Leftovers can be saved in a sealed container to be microwaved later.

Per 1-ounce serving (2 strips): 118 calories, 13 g protein, 5 g carbohydrate, 2 g sugar, 6 g fat, 44% calories from fat, 3 g fiber, 434 mg sodium

Grilled Breakfast Tofu

MAKES 2 SERVINGS

With a texture almost identical to egg white, tofu is a common part of a Japanese breakfast and is loaded with protein. This simple recipe adds savory flavors.

½ block (approximately 7 ounces) firm tofu

Vegetable oil spray (if not using a nonstick pan)

½ teaspoon ground ginger

1 tablespoon nutritional yeast

1 teaspoon low-sodium soy sauce

Remove the tofu from the pack, rinse, and squeeze out any extra water. Cut thin (¼-inch-thick) slices from the block. Place the slices in a nonstick frying pan (or a pan prepared with a whiff of vegetable oil spray) and cook over medium heat for 5 to 7 minutes. Turn, and cook another 5 to 7 minutes, or until golden. Transfer to a serving plate and top with ginger, nutritional yeast, and soy sauce.

Note: If you prefer, the tofu can also be served without cooking, at room temperature. Simply rinse it, slice it, and add the toppings.

Per 3½-ounce serving (½ of recipe): 124 calories, 15 g protein, 6 g carbohydrate, 1 g sugar, 6 g fat, 39% calories from fat, 2 g fiber, 113 mg sodium

Breakfast Apple Crisp

MAKES 4 TO 6 SERVINGS

APPLE FILLING:

4 red apples, cored and diced

1 teaspoon cornstarch

1 teaspoon cinnamon

3 tablespoons sugar

CRISP TOPPING

1 cup quick oats

1 teaspoon cinnamon

3 tablespoons maple syrup

Preheat the oven to 350°F. Lightly spray a 9-inch glass pie plate with cooking spray.

Place the apples in a large bowl. Add the cornstarch, cinnamon, and sugar. Stir to evenly coat all the apples. Transfer the apples to the glass pie plate.

In a separate bowl, combine all the crisp topping ingredients. Evenly spread the topping over the apples and bake for 1 hour. Serve warm, room temperature, or chilled.

Per serving (¼ of recipe): 252 calories, 3 g protein, 60 g carbohydrate, 37 g sugar, 2 g fat, 6% calories from fat, 7 g fiber, 5 mg sodium

Recipe by Christine Waltermyer

Banana Blueberry Smoothie

MAKES 2 SERVINGS

2 cups frozen blueberries

2 ripe bananas, sliced

1 cup almond milk

1 cup ice

¼ cup maple syrup

Place all ingredients in a blender and process until smooth. If you like it less thick, you can replace some of the ice with an equal amount of almond milk.

Per serving (½ of recipe): 353 calories, 3 g protein, 85 g carbohydrate, 61 g sugar, 3 g fat, 7% calories from fat, 10 g fiber, 86 mg sodium

Recipe by Christine Waltermyer

Chia Breakfast Parfait

MAKES 3 SMALL MASON JARS

2 cups unsweetened vanilla almond milk

½ cup chia seeds

3 tablespoons maple syrup

½ teaspoon vanilla extract

2 cups mixed berries (blueberries, strawberries, raspberries, boysenberries)

Fresh mint sprigs

In a medium bowl, combine the almond milk, chia seeds, maple syrup, and vanilla extract. Whisk to combine. Cover the bowl with plastic wrap and refrigerate for 6 hours or overnight.

The next day, spoon the chia pudding and mixed berries in alternating layers into three small mason jars. Finish with a layer of berries and top with fresh mint sprigs.

Per serving (⅓ of recipe): 246 calories, 6 g protein, 36 g carbohydrate, 18 g sugar, 10 g fat, 35% calories from fat, 13 g fiber, 121 mg sodium

Recipe by Christine Waltermyer

SALADS

Colorful Quinoa Salad

MAKES 8 SERVINGS

½ red onion, chopped

2 tablespoons freshly squeezed lemon juice

2 tablespoons apple cider vinegar

⅛ teaspoon salt

12 ounces frozen shelled edamame

1¼ cups frozen corn

1½ cups cooked and cooled quinoa

1 red bell pepper, chopped

½ teaspoon chili powder

½ teaspoon dried thyme

¼ teaspoon freshly ground black pepper

Place the onion in a small bowl and add the lemon juice, apple cider vinegar, and salt. Mix well and set aside to marinate for 5 to 10 minutes (reserve marinade).

In a medium saucepan, combine the edamame and corn with ½ cup water. Bring to a boil and cook for 4 minutes. Drain in a strainer and run cold water over the vegetables to cool them.

In a large salad bowl, combine the cooked quinoa, marinated onions with lemon juice and vinegar, edamame and corn, bell pepper, chili powder, thyme, and black pepper. Toss gently to mix. Adjust seasonings to taste.

Per ¾-cup serving (⅛ of recipe): 123 calories, 8 g protein, 18 g carbohydrate, 3 g sugar, 3 g fat, 22% calories from fat, 4 g fiber, 47 mg sodium

Recipe by Rose Saltalamacchia

Pizza Pasta Salad

MAKES 12 (1-CUP) SERVINGS

16 ounces dry pasta

1 (15-ounce) can chickpeas or cannellini beans, drained and
rinsed

1 (15-ounce) can kidney beans, drained and rinsed

1 large green bell pepper, chopped

1 large yellow or orange bell pepper, chopped

1 cup dry (not oil-packed) sun-dried tomatoes, thinly sliced (see
note)

½ cup diced red onion

½ cup pitted black olives (measured whole, then sliced)

¾ cup fat-free or light Italian dressing

1 teaspoon dried oregano

¼ cup toasted pine nuts (optional)

Cook the pasta according to the package directions. Meanwhile, toss the remaining ingredients in a large bowl, reserving 1 tablespoon pine nuts, if using. When the pasta is cooked, rinse with cold water, drain, and immediately add to the bowl with the other ingredients. Toss gently. Top with the remaining pine nuts, if using.

Note: If the sun-dried tomatoes are not moist, soak in hot water for 20 minutes and drain before adding to the pasta salad.

Per 1-cup serving (¹/₁₂ of recipe): 255 calories, 11 g protein, 47 g carbohydrate, 6 g sugar, 3 g fat, 9% calories from fat, 6 g fiber, 298 mg sodium

Recipe by Lee Crosby

Mediterranean Lentils

This colorful salad is healthful and easy to make.

1 cup dry green lentils

1 cup chopped tomato

1 cup peeled and chopped cucumber

1 cup chopped orange or red bell pepper (cut into small cubes)

½ cup chopped carrot (cut into small cubes)

2 garlic cloves, finely chopped

¼ cup chopped olives

1 tablespoon chopped fresh basil, or 1 teaspoon dried basil

¼ cup balsamic vinegar

⅛ teaspoon salt

Black pepper, to taste

Clean the lentils, making sure they have no stones, and pour into a large pot of water. Boil gently for 20 minutes, or until tender. Strain and let cool on a tray in the refrigerator. In a large bowl, mix the cooled lentils, tomato, cucumber, bell pepper, carrot, garlic, olives, basil, and balsamic vinegar. Season with salt and black pepper. Serve the salad cold, either alone or accompanied by a lettuce salad.

Per serving (¼ of recipe): 210 calories, 13 g protein, 37 g carbo-hydrate, 7 g sugar, 2 g fat, 7% calories from fat, 10 g fiber, 158 mg sodium

Recipe by Dora Stone

Vegan Caesar Salad

MAKES 6 SERVINGS

DRESSING:

½ cup soft silken tofu

2 tablespoons water

1 tablespoon lemon juice

1 tablespoon red wine vinegar

1 garlic clove, coarsely chopped

2 teaspoons Dijon mustard

1 teaspoon capers

½ teaspoon vegetarian Worcestershire sauce

Black pepper, to taste

SALAD:

3 romaine lettuce hearts, washed and torn into bite-size pieces

6 tablespoons toasted pumpkin seeds

3 tablespoons superfine almond flour

Place all dressing ingredients in a blender and process until smooth. Adjust to taste.

Just before serving the salad, combine the romaine lettuce, toasted pumpkin seeds, and desired amount of dressing. Toss to evenly coat the lettuce with the dressing. Sprinkle with the almond flour and toss again before serving.

Per serving (⅙ of recipe): 94 calories, 6 g protein, 6 g carbohydrate, 2 g sugar, 6 g fat, 57% calories from fat, 3 g fiber, 90 mg sodium

Recipe by Christine Waltermyer

Fruity Spinach Salad

MAKES 4 SERVINGS

6 cups baby spinach, lightly packed

1 red or yellow apple, cored and diced (skin on)

4 tablespoons diced red onion

½ cup pomegranate seeds

1 cup sliced strawberries

¼ cup walnuts, pecans, or sliced almonds

RASPBERRY VINAIGRETTE DRESSING:

¼ cup nondairy plain yogurt

2 tablespoons apple cider vinegar

¼ cup all-fruit raspberry jam

2 teaspoons Dijon mustard

Pinch of sea salt

Place all salad ingredients in a large salad bowl. In a small bowl, whisk together all dressing ingredients. Just before serving, pour dressing over the salad and toss.

Per serving (1/4 of recipe): 168 calories, 4 g protein, 28 g carbohydrate, 20 g sugar, 6 g fat, 30% calories from fat, 5 g fiber, 176 mg sodium

Recipe by Christine Waltermyer

SOUPS

Minestrone

MAKES 8 SERVINGS

½ onion, chopped

6 cups low-sodium vegetable broth, divided

4 garlic cloves, finely chopped

1 cup diced carrots

2 celery stalks, sliced

2 potatoes, peeled and diced

1 (28-ounce) can diced tomatoes

1 zucchini, chopped

2 teaspoons dried basil

1 tablespoon dried parsley

¼ teaspoon sea salt

Black pepper, to taste

1 (15-ounce) can kidney beans, drained and rinsed

1 cup dry macaroni noodles

½ cup frozen lima beans

1½ cups fresh chopped spinach, or ½ cup frozen chopped spinach

Sauté the onion in ¼ cup of the vegetable broth on medium-low heat for 4 minutes. Add the garlic and sauté for 3 more minutes. Add the carrots, celery, potatoes, tomatoes, and remaining vegetable broth. Increase the heat to medium-high to bring to a boil. Reduce the heat to medium-low and simmer, covered, for 20 minutes. Then add the zucchini, basil, parsley, sea salt, black pepper, kidney beans, macaroni, and lima beans. Increase the heat to medium-high to bring back to a boil. Boil for 1 minute, then reduce the heat to simmer on low, covered, for 8 more minutes. Add the spinach and cook for 3 more minutes.

Per serving (1/8 of recipe): 203 calories, 9 g protein, 41 g carbohydrate, 7 g sugar, 1 g fat, 6% calories from fat, 7 g fiber, 396 mg sodium

Recipe by Noah Kauffman

Corn Chowder

MAKES 8 SERVINGS

1 yellow onion, chopped

1 red bell pepper, chopped

2 garlic cloves, minced

4½ cups low-sodium vegetable broth

2 cups chopped potatoes

2 tablespoons all-purpose flour

2 cups unsweetened almond milk (or other nondairy milk)

2 cups frozen corn

Black pepper, to taste

In a large pot, sauté the onion and bell pepper over medium-high heat, adding small amounts of water to keep the vegetables from sticking, for 8 to 10 minutes, until the onion is soft and translucent. Add the garlic and sauté for another 30 seconds. Add the vegetable broth and potatoes.

In a separate bowl, whisk the flour with the almond milk until there are no lumps. Add the flour and almond milk mixture to the pot. When the soup comes to a boil, turn the heat down to medium and cook for 15 to 20 minutes, or until the potatoes are fork-tender.

Add the frozen corn when there are 5 minutes left of cooking time. Add black pepper to taste.

Per serving (1 cup): 97 calories, 3 g protein, 21 g carbohydrate, 3 g sugar, 1 g fat, 10% calories from fat, 2 g fiber, 122 mg sodium

Recipe by Karen Smith

Pasta e Fagioli

MAKES 8 SERVINGS

4 cups low-sodium vegetable broth

1 small onion, chopped

6 garlic cloves, finely chopped

2 (15-ounce) cans Great Northern beans, drained

1 (6-ounce) can tomato paste

1 (28-ounce) can low-sodium crushed tomatoes

16 ounces dry farfalle pasta

Black pepper, to taste

2 tablespoons fresh chopped basil

Heat 2 tablespoons of the vegetable broth in a large pot. Sauté the onion and garlic for 7 minutes. Add to the pot the remaining broth and the beans, tomato paste, and crushed tomatoes, along with their liquid. Heat on high until the soup boils. Add the pasta, cover, and cook on medium heat until the pasta is al dente (about 14 minutes). Stir the pasta occasionally while cooking. Season with black pepper to taste. Add the fresh basil during the last 3 minutes of cooking.

Per serving (⅛ of recipe): 393 calories, 18 g protein, 76 g carbohydrate, 7 g sugar, 2 g fat, 4% calories from fat, 10 g fiber, 518 mg sodium

Recipe by Noah Kauffman

Pearled Barley Soup

MAKES 6 SERVINGS

This thick soup is a typical daily dish in Colombia.

  1 white onion, chopped

  4 garlic cloves, finely chopped

  1 scallion, thinly sliced

  ¾ cup dry pearled barley, rinsed

  10 cups low-sodium vegetable broth

  1 bay leaf

  1 sprig fresh cilantro

  1 cup chopped carrots

  2 cups peeled and chopped potatoes

  1½ cups frozen green peas

  Black pepper, to taste

  1 avocado, sliced

  1 tomato, chopped

Heat a large pot over medium heat. Add the onion and stir and sweat for 6 to 7 minutes, or until the onion is tender and translucent. If it starts to stick to the pan, add a little water or vegetable broth. Add the garlic and scallion and cook for 2 more minutes. Add the barley, vegetable broth, bay leaf, cilantro, carrots, and potatoes. Bring to a boil over medium-high heat. Reduce the heat to low and simmer, covered, for 25 minutes or until the barley, carrots, and potatoes are tender. Add the green peas and cook for 5 more minutes. Season with black pepper to taste. Serve with slices of avocado and chopped tomato.

Note: If you begin to cook the onion at a low temperature, it releases its natural juices, obviating the need for cooking oil.

Per serving (⅙ of recipe): 349 calories, 11 g protein, 66 g carbohydrate, 9 g sugar, 6 g fat, 16% calories from fat, 14 g fiber, 270 mg sodium

Recipe by Dora Stone

Quick Black Bean Chili

(6 SERVINGS)

It gets no easier than this. Everyone loves this dish, and it's even better the next day!

1 (25-ounce) can low-sodium black beans, drained, liquid reserved (see note)

1¾ cups homemade salsa, or 1 (16-ounce) jar or container salsa (mild, medium, or hot, depending on preference)

1 cup frozen corn

2 teaspoons chili powder

½ teaspoon ground cumin

Black pepper, to taste

Squeeze of fresh lime juice (optional)

Chopped fresh cilantro (optional)

Mix the drained beans, salsa, corn, chili powder, and cumin in a soup pot. Add enough reserved bean liquid to achieve the desired consistency. Heat over medium heat for 20 minutes, stirring occasionally. Season with black pepper. Add the lime juice and cilantro, if desired, before serving.

VARIATIONS: To speed the cooking time, defrost the corn under cold running water before combining the ingredients. Alternatively, the ingredients can be mixed in a slow cooker and cooked on high for 75 minutes or on low for 8 or more hours. (Add additional liquid, either vegetable broth or water, if needed.)

Note: Dried black beans that have been soaked and cooked may be used in place of canned beans. To equal 1 (25-ounce) can, use 2½ cups of cooked beans and cover with cooking liquid to equal a total of 3 cups.

Per serving (⅙ of recipe): 147 calories, 8 g protein, 29 g carbohydrate, 2 g sugar, 1 g fat, 5% calories from fat, 10 g fiber, 258 mg sodium

Recipe by Caroline Trapp

Potato Leek Soup

MAKES 4 SERVINGS

This rich-tasting soup is surprisingly low in fat, so go ahead and enjoy a steaming bowl.

4 leeks, white and light green parts, split lengthwise, washed, and sliced

1 teaspoon dried thyme

1½ pounds potatoes, peeled and diced

4 to 5 cups low-sodium vegetable broth

Freshly ground black pepper

1 tablespoon minced fresh parsley, for garnish

In a large saucepan, heat 2 tablespoons water over medium-low heat. Add the leeks and thyme and cook, stirring, for 10 minutes. Add the potatoes and 4 cups of vegetable broth, raise the heat to medium-high, and bring to a gentle boil. Reduce the heat to low, cover, and simmer for 30 minutes. Remove from the heat and, using an immersion blender, puree at least half or all of the soup, depending on how smooth you like it. Add a little more broth if the soup is too thick. Season with black pepper to taste. Serve hot, garnished with the parsley.

Per serving (¼ of recipe): 183 calories, 4 g protein, 42 g carbohydrate, 5 g sugar, 1 g fat, 3% calories from fat, 5 g fiber, 156 mg sodium

Recipe by Christine Waltermyer

SANDWICHES AND MAIN DISHES

Super-Quick Hummus

MAKES 10 SERVINGS

2 cups canned or cooked chickpeas

1 garlic clove, finely chopped

¼ cup tahini

Juice of 2 lemons

¼ cup finely chopped fresh parsley

¼ cup chopped green onions

½ cup water

¼ teaspoon black pepper, or to taste

⅛ teaspoon salt, or to taste

Blend all the ingredients in a food processor, adding more water, if needed, for a smooth consistency.

Serve as a dip, as a sandwich filling in pita bread, or on sandwich bread with chopped tomatoes, lettuce, or sprouts.

Tip: For a lower-fat hummus, reduce the tahini as desired.

Per 3-tablespoon serving (¹/₁₀ of recipe): 83 calories, 3 g protein, 9 g carbohydrate, 4 g fat, 42% calories from fat, 3 g fiber, 119 mg sodium

Hummus Wrap

MAKES 2 SERVINGS

2 large fat-free tortillas

3 cups mixed greens

1 cup shredded carrots

1 cup shredded red cabbage

HUMMUS:

1 (15-ounce) can low-sodium chickpeas, or 1½ cups cooked chickpeas

2 to 3 tablespoons lemon juice

2 green onions, sliced, or 1 garlic clove, minced

⅛ teaspoon sea salt (optional)

3 tablespoons water

Place all hummus ingredients in a food processor and blend until smooth. Adjust seasonings to taste.

Heat the tortillas by placing them in a hot skillet for a few minutes on each side. Then spread a generous amount of hummus on each one, top with mixed greens, carrots, and red cabbage. Wrap/roll up tightly and enjoy!

Per serving (½ of recipe): 394 calories, 16 g protein, 67 g carbohydrate, 13 g sugar, 8 g fat, 18% calories from fat, 15 g fiber, 449 mg sodium

Recipe by Christine Waltermyer

Chickpea "Tuna" Salad

MAKES 2 TO 4 SERVINGS

1 (15-ounce) can low-sodium chickpeas, drained and rinsed

¼ cup commercial garlic hummus

1 teaspoon Dijon mustard

2 tablespoons chopped onion

2 tablespoons pickle relish

Black pepper, to taste

Optional: 1 teaspoon dulse or kelp granules (finely ground sea
        vegetable condiment available at natural food stores)

Place the chickpeas in a large bowl and partially mash with a potato masher. The idea is to keep a little texture. Add the garlic hummus, Dijon mustard, chopped onion, pickle relish, black pepper, and optional dulse or kelp granules. Adjust seasonings to taste.

Serve the Chickpea "Tuna" Salad with crudités or use it as a sandwich filling with toasted whole grain bread, sliced tomato, and shredded carrots.

Per serving (½ of recipe): 269 calories, 12 g protein, 43 g carbohydrate, 11 g sugar, 7 g fat, 21% calories from fat, 11 g fiber, 326 mg sodium

Recipe by Christine Waltermyer

Lasagna with Cashew Tofu Ricotta

MAKES 8 SERVINGS

9 dry lasagna noodles

2 (12-ounce) packages silken tofu (extra-firm)

¾ cup cashews

2 teaspoons dried basil

2 tablespoons lemon juice

24 ounces low-sodium commercial pasta sauce

Preheat the oven to 350°F.

Boil the lasagna noodles according to the package directions, then drain and rinse with cold water. Combine the tofu, cashews, basil, and lemon juice in a food processor or blender and process until smooth. Layer in a lightly oiled lasagna pan: pasta sauce, 3 cooked noodles, and tofu-cashew mixture. Repeat with another layer of sauce, 3 more noodles, and tofu-cashew mixture. Top with more sauce, the remaining 3 noodles, and the remaining sauce. Bake uncovered for 20 to 30 minutes.

Per serving (⅛ of recipe): 267 calories, 13 g protein, 32 g carbohydrate, 7 g sugar, 10 g fat, 32% calories from fat, 3 g fiber, 59 mg sodium

Recipe by Noah Kauffman

Easy Stuffed Peppers

MAKES 4 SERVINGS

1 cup dry brown rice

1 yellow onion, chopped

2 garlic cloves, finely chopped

2 tablespoons chili powder

2 teaspoons ground cumin

1 (15-ounce) can low-sodium black beans, drained and rinsed

Black pepper, to taste

1¾ cups homemade salsa, or 1 (16-ounce) jar salsa

4 bell peppers, any color

Preheat the oven to 350°F. Cook the rice as directed on the package.

Heat a large saucepan over medium heat. Add the onion and stir frequently. You may need to add water or low-sodium vegetable broth in small increments to prevent the onion from sticking or burning. Sauté for about 5 minutes. Add the garlic and sauté for 1 more minute. Add the chili powder and cumin to the onion and garlic and stir for about 30 seconds. Add the black beans, black pepper, and half the salsa. Once the mixture begins to boil, reduce the heat to low and let simmer for 5 to 10 minutes.

Cut off the tops of the bell peppers and remove the membrane and seeds. If needed, slice off a thin piece from the bottoms of the bell peppers so they can stand upright in a rectangular baking dish.

Put the remaining salsa in the bottom of the baking dish. Place the peppers inside the baking dish. Once the rice is cooked, add it to the bean and salsa mixture, and stir to combine. With a spoon, fill each pepper with the mixture. Cover with tin foil and bake for 45 to 50 minutes.

Per serving (1 pepper): 367 calories, 13 g protein, 75 g carbohydrate, 8 g sugar, 3 g fat, 7% calories from fat, 14 g fiber, 474 mg sodium

Recipe by Karen Smith

Pasta Bowl with Beans and Greens

MAKES 4 SERVINGS

This pasta dish is packed with plenty of vegetables and beans, making it more satisfying than and just as delicious as a traditional Italian pasta marinara.

8 ounces dry whole-grain pasta

2 cups thinly sliced white button or baby portobello mushrooms

1 (6- to 9-ounce) container prewashed fresh kale, chopped (or spinach, collard greens, frozen kale, etc. See note)

2 zucchini or yellow squash, spiralized or thinly sliced

2 cups commercial pasta sauce

1 (15-ounce) can no-salt-added or reduced-sodium white beans, drained and rinsed

¼ cup nutritional yeast

OPTIONAL FLAVOR ADDITIONS:

1 (14-ounce) can water-packed artichoke hearts or hearts of palm

4 garlic cloves, finely chopped

½ teaspoon cayenne pepper

¼ cup julienned fresh basil, for garnish

Cook the pasta al dente according to the package directions.

Sauté the mushrooms in a pan on medium heat using 1 tablespoon water to prevent sticking. After 3 minutes, add the kale and any optional flavor additions. Cook for 2 minutes, then add the zucchini. Cook for 3 more minutes. Remove from heat and set aside.

Once the pasta is finished cooking and drained, add it back to its original pan and stir in the pasta sauce, beans, and nutritional yeast. Cook on low heat for 1 to 2 minutes to warm the sauce.

Gently fold in the sautéed vegetables to the pot. Serve warm and with additional nutritional yeast or julienned basil on top, if desired.

Note: If using other types of leafy greens, you will need to adjust the cooking time. Cook collard greens for 5 to 10 minutes, spinach or frozen kale for only 1 minute.

Per serving (¼ of recipe): 452 calories, 26 g protein, 87 g carbohydrate, 13 g sugar, 4 g fat, 8% calories from fat, 18 g fiber, 393 mg sodium

Recipe by Maggie Neola

Spaghetti Alfredo

MAKES 2 SERVINGS

1 onion, chopped

3 garlic cloves, finely chopped

1 tablespoon low-sodium vegetable broth

¾ cup almond milk or cashew milk

Pinch of salt

1 cup chopped cauliflower

1 tablespoon nutritional yeast

½ tablespoon lemon juice

4 ounces dry whole wheat spaghetti or 3 to 4 cups cooked spaghetti squash*

Sauté the onion and garlic in the vegetable broth until golden brown, 3 to 4 minutes. Add the almond milk and bring it to a boil. Add the salt and cauliflower and cook until the cauliflower is soft, about 7 minutes. Transfer to a blender and add the nutritional yeast and lemon juice. Blend until smooth.

Cook the pasta al dente according to the package directions. Drain, and pour the pasta into the pan with the sauce. Stir and serve.

*To prepare the spaghetti squash: Preheat the oven to 350°F. Carefully halve a raw spaghetti squash and remove the seeds with a large spoon. Place the halves on a baking sheet facing up. Sprinkle with black pepper to taste. Bake for about an hour, or until the inside strands can be easily pulled out with a fork. Use the fork to remove all "spaghetti" strands. Serve with Alfredo sauce above.

Per serving with whole wheat spaghetti (½ of recipe): 315 calories, 14 g protein, 62 g carbohydrate, 7 g sugar, 4 g fat, 11% calories from fat, 9 g fiber, 226 mg sodium

Recipe by Hana Kahleova

Mixed Vegetable Stir-Fry

MAKES 4 SERVINGS

CHINESE BROWN SAUCE:

½ cup low-sodium vegetable broth

½ cup apple juice

2 tablespoons low-sodium soy sauce

4 garlic cloves, minced

2 teaspoons fresh ginger root, peeled and minced

1 tablespoon maple syrup

2 teaspoons apple cider vinegar

Black pepper, to taste

MIX TOGETHER SEPARATELY:

1 tablespoon cornstarch

2 tablespoons water

STIR-FRY:

¼ cup low-sodium vegetable broth

1 onion, sliced

2 cups sliced button mushrooms

1 red bell pepper, cut into strips

Pinch of sea salt

3 carrots, sliced diagonally

1 cup green beans, trimmed and cut in half on a diagonal

2 cups broccoli spears

1 cup snow peas, trimmed

Place all Chinese Brown Sauce ingredients, except the cornstarch and water, into a small saucepan. Separately, mix the cornstarch and water together until smooth. Add to the saucepan and slowly heat, while whisking, over medium heat. The sauce is finished once it thickens to desired consistency. If it gets too thick, you can dilute with a little more vegetable broth. If it needs to be thicker, you can add more diluted cornstarch. Adjust seasoning to taste.

To make the stir-fry, heat a large skillet or wok over medium-high heat. Add two or three tablespoons of the vegetable broth and heat briefly. Add the onion, mushrooms, bell pepper, and sea salt. Cook and stir for a few minutes. Add the carrots and green beans, cover, and cook a few minutes longer. Add a little more vegetable broth if the vegetables begin to stick to the skillet. Add the broccoli and snow peas. Cook until the vegetables are brightly colored and crisp-tender. Add as much of the sauce as you wish and serve over Perfect Brown Rice (page 136).

Per serving (¼ of recipe): 115 calories, 4 g protein, 25 g carbohydrate, 13 g sugar, 1 g fat, 5% calories from fat, 5 g fiber, 429 mg sodium

Recipe by Christine Waltermyer

GRAINS AND VEGETABLES

Perfect Brown Rice

MAKES 3 CUPS

It's great to get to know brown rice. Some of the healthiest, slimmest, longest-lived people on the planet live in rural Asia and make rice their staple. In this recipe, the rice is briefly toasted and then cooked like pasta, without allowing too much water to be absorbed. It will be the best rice you've ever tasted.

1 cup dry short-grain brown rice
3 cups water

Place the rice in a saucepan, rinse with water, then drain away the water. Place the pan on high heat and stir the rice until dry, about 2 minutes. Add the water. Bring to a boil, then simmer until the rice is thoroughly cooked but still retains just a hint of crunchiness—about 40 minutes. Drain off the remaining water. Do not cook the rice until all the water is absorbed. Top with soy sauce, sesame seeds, cooked vegetables, beans, or lentils, if desired.

Per ½-cup serving: 115 calories, 2.7 g protein, 24 g carbohydrate, 0.4 g sugar, 1 g fat, 7% calories from fat, 3 g fiber, 5 mg sodium

Polenta

MAKES 4 TO 6 SERVINGS

Polenta is an Italian staple that is as healthful as it is simple. Italian singing star Naif Hérin grew up in the Italian Alps and shared her family recipe with us.

5 cups water

1 cup cornmeal

½ teaspoon salt

Combine all the ingredients in a saucepan. Bring to a boil, whisking. Reduce the heat to simmer on low heat for 60 minutes, stirring occasionally with a whisk.

Serving suggestions: Top with mushrooms, tomatoes, or other ingredients. The Mushroom Ragout (recipe below) is especially delicious with polenta.

Per serving (¼ of recipe): 145 calories, 3 g protein, 31 g carbohydrate, 1 g sugar, 1 g fat, 4% calories from fat, 2 g fiber, 306 mg sodium

Recipe by Naif Hérin

Mushroom Ragout

MAKES 4 TO 6 SERVINGS

This is a delicious topping for polenta.

1 cup low-sodium vegetable broth

1 onion, chopped

4 garlic cloves, finely chopped

1 cup chopped carrots

2 pounds sliced mixed fresh mushrooms (shiitakes, button, cremini, etc.)

2 teaspoons fresh thyme leaves, or 1 teaspoon dried thyme

½ cup tomato puree

2 tablespoons low-sodium soy sauce

Black pepper, to taste

¼ cup chopped fresh parsley, for garnish

Heat ¼ cup of the vegetable broth in a large sauté pan over medium heat. Add the onion and cook for 5 minutes, stirring occasionally. Add the garlic, carrots, mushrooms, and thyme. Cover and cook for 8 more minutes, stirring occasionally. Add the remaining ¾ cup vegetable broth, tomato puree, and soy sauce. Stir and bring to a boil over medium-high heat. Reduce the heat to simmer on low, covered, for 30 minutes. Season with black pepper and serve hot. Garnish with the parsley.

Per serving (¼ of recipe): 89 calories, 6 g protein, 18 g carbohydrate, 8 g sugar, 1 g fat, 9% calories from fat, 5 g fiber, 405 mg sodium

Recipe by Christine Waltermyer

Loaded Baked Sweet Potato

MAKES 4 SERVINGS

The ultimate fast food!

- 4 medium sweet potatoes
- 2 cups cooked black beans, or 1 (15-ounce) can black beans
- 1 cup salsa
- ½ cup chopped fresh cilantro
- ¼ cup mashed avocado or dry-roasted pepitas (pumpkin seeds) (optional)

Wash the sweet potatoes. Pierce each potato 4 to 5 times with a fork and bake in the oven or microwave.

<u>Oven</u>: Preheat the oven to 400°F. Place the potatoes on a rimmed baking sheet lined with foil or parchment paper. Bake 45 to 75 minutes, or until tender.

<u>Microwave</u>: Place the potatoes in a microwave-safe dish with ½ cup water. Cover loosely with a lid or plastic wrap. Microwave for

10 minutes. Carefully turn the potatoes over. Microwave another 10 to 12 minutes, or until the potatoes are tender.

Once cooked, split the potatoes and top each potato with black beans, salsa, cilantro, and mashed avocado or pepitas, if using.

Note: Other tasty toppings include corn (fresh or thawed from frozen), chopped tomatoes, and sliced green onions.

Per potato: 235 calories, 11 g protein, 48 g carbohydrate, 11 g sugar, 1 g fat, 3% calories from fat, 13 g fiber, 503 mg sodium

Recipe by Lee Crosby

Baked and Breaded Cauliflower
MAKES 4 SERVINGS

1 head cauliflower, separated into florets

1 cup almond milk

½ cup whole wheat flour

Pinch of salt

3 garlic cloves, finely chopped

Preheat the oven to 350°F. Line a baking sheet with parchment paper.

Cook the cauliflower in boiling water for 5 to 10 minutes. In a small bowl, mix the almond milk with the flour, salt, and garlic. Dip the cooked cauliflower into the mixture and place on the baking sheet. Bake for 30 to 40 minutes, until golden.

Per serving (¼ of recipe): 100 calories, 5 g protein, 19 g carbohydrate, 5 g sugar, 2 g fat, 14% calories from fat, 5 g fiber, 133 mg sodium

Recipe by Hana Kahleova

Garlic Sautéed Baby Bok Choy

MAKES 4 SERVINGS

¼ cup vegetable broth

1 pound baby bok choy, rinsed and halved lengthwise

3 garlic cloves, minced

1 tablespoon low-sodium soy sauce

Crushed red pepper flakes (optional)

2 teaspoons fresh lemon juice or rice vinegar

Heat the vegetable broth in a large pan over high heat. Add the baby bok choy, garlic, and soy sauce. Cover and cook for 2 minutes. Remove the lid and turn the bok choy to cook the other side. If using the optional crushed red pepper flakes, add them now. If your vegetable broth has evaporated, you can add another splash to keep the pan from going dry. Cook for another 2 minutes, or until desired tenderness. Baby bok choy is delicious when the leaves are wilted and the stems are crisp-tender. Sprinkle with the lemon juice or rice vinegar just before serving.

Per serving (¼ of recipe): 19 calories, 2 g protein, 3 g carbohydrate, 1 g sugar, 0.2 g fat, 9% calories from fat, 1 g fiber, 218 mg sodium

Recipe by Christine Waltermyer

DESSERTS

Manhattan Tricolor

MAKES 2 SERVINGS

The blue, orange, and white of the New York City flag come alive in this simple, healthful way to finish a meal. The Bronx version of the flag adds a helpful motto for anyone tempted by unhealthful desserts: *Ne cede malis* (Yield not to evil).

6 ounces fresh blueberries

1 mango or papaya, chopped

1 banana, sliced

1 tablespoon whole almonds

Combine all ingredients and serve immediately.

Tip: If slicing a mango seems like a daunting task, you will find mango slicers online that allow you to remove the seed and peel the skin in seconds.

Per serving (½ of recipe): 228 calories, 4 g protein, 52 g carbohydrate, 39 g sugar, 3 g fat, 12% calories from fat, 7 g fiber, 3 mg sodium

Raspberry Fudgy Brownies

MAKES 16 BROWNIES

2 (15-ounce) cans black beans, drained and rinsed

1 cup pitted dates

1 cup all-fruit raspberry jam

2 teaspoons pure vanilla extract

¼ cup plus 2 tablespoons whole wheat pastry flour

1 cup unsweetened cocoa powder

¼ teaspoon sea salt

½ cup mini chocolate chips or ½ cup raspberry all-fruit jam, for topping (optional)

Preheat the oven to 350°F. Line an 8 x 8-inch baking pan with parchment paper.

Combine the black beans, dates, jam, and vanilla in a food processor. Blend until smooth. Add the flour, cocoa powder, and sea salt and blend again. Pour into the prepared pan and smooth the top with moist hands. If desired, sprinkle evenly with the chocolate chips or spread with the raspberry jam.

Bake for 30 minutes. Remove from the oven and cool completely. Use the parchment paper to lift the brownies out of the pan. Cut into 16 squares. Refrigerate for up to 1 week, stored in a covered container.

Per serving (1/16 of recipe): 136 calories, 5 g protein, 30 g carbohydrate, 14 g sugar, 1 g total fat, 7% calories from fat, 7 g fiber, 110 mg sodium

Recipe by Christine Waltermyer

Mixed Berry Sorbet

MAKES 2 CUPS

½ cup almond milk

1 cup frozen mixed berries

1 cup frozen sliced bananas

¼ cup maple syrup (optional)

Place the almond milk in a food processor or high-speed blender. Add the berries, bananas, and maple syrup, if using. Blend until smooth.

Place the mixture in a plastic container and freeze for 30 minutes. Stir the sorbet with a fork and freeze for 30 more minutes, or until it reaches the desired consistency. Using an ice cream scoop, serve the sorbet.

Any leftover sorbet will firm up quite a bit, so remove it from the freezer 15 minutes before serving to soften it.

Per ½-cup serving (¼ of recipe): 60 calories, 1 g protein, 15 g carbohydrate, 8 g sugar, 0.5 g fat, 7% calories from fat, 2 g fiber, 20 mg sodium

Recipe by Christine Waltermyer

Chai-Spiced Pudding

MAKES 2 SERVINGS

⅓ cup millet, rinsed

2 cups almond milk

3 tablespoons maple syrup or agave nectar

2 tablespoons dried currants or raisins

1 teaspoon pure vanilla extract

1 teaspoon ground cinnamon

½ teaspoon ground ginger

¼ teaspoon ground cardamom

¼ teaspoon ground allspice

Pinch of ground cloves

In a medium saucepan, combine the millet and almond milk. Bring to a boil uncovered, over medium-high heat. Reduce the heat to simmer on low, and cook, covered, for 25 minutes, or until the millet is soft and creamy. Stir occasionally as it cooks.

Add the maple syrup, currants, vanilla, and spices and cook for 5 more minutes. Serve warm or chilled. If the pudding becomes too firm when chilled, add more almond milk to create the desired consistency.

Per serving (½ of recipe): 297 calories, 5 g protein, 61 g carbohydrate, 32 g sugar, 4 g fat, 11% calories from fat, 5 g fiber, 160 mg sodium

Recipe by Christine Waltermyer

Spiced Apple Gel

1½ cups no-sugar-added apple juice

2 tablespoons maple syrup

Pinch of sea salt

1 cup chopped apple (with or without peel)

1 tablespoon plus 1 teaspoon agar-agar flakes, or 1 teaspoon
agar-agar powder (see note)

½ teaspoon cornstarch

½ teaspoon ground cinnamon

Place 1¼ cups of the apple juice in a medium saucepan with the maple syrup, sea salt, and apple. Add the agar-agar flakes. Whisk to combine. Bring to a boil, uncovered, over high heat, whisking occasionally. Reduce the heat to simmer on medium-low for 10 minutes, or until the agar-agar flakes are dissolved.

Place the remaining ¼ cup apple juice in a small bowl and add the cornstarch. Mix well, then stir this into the apple juice–maple syrup mixture in the saucepan. Add the cinnamon and stir with a whisk to thoroughly incorporate.

Remove from the heat and pour the apple dessert into serving bowls and cool to room temperature. Refrigerate for an hour or until firm. Serve cool.

Note: You can find agar-agar flakes at most health food stores or online. You can experiment using slightly more or less agar-agar depending on how firm you like your apple dessert to be.

Per ½-cup serving: 87 calories, 0.3 g protein, 22 g carbohydrate, 18 g sugar, 0.2 g fat, 2% calories from fat, 1 g fiber, 81 mg sodium

Recipe by Christine Waltermyer

Banana Bread

1½ cups mashed bananas (about 4 large bananas)

1 cup sugar

¼ cup nondairy milk

1 teaspoon vanilla extract

1 teaspoon lemon juice or apple cider vinegar

1 cup unbleached white flour

1 cup whole wheat or spelt flour

1 teaspoon baking soda

½ teaspoon baking powder

½ teaspoon sea salt

1 teaspoon cinnamon

⅛ teaspoon nutmeg

Preheat the oven to 350°F. In a large bowl, mix together the mashed bananas, sugar, nondairy milk, vanilla, and lemon juice. In a separate bowl, combine the flours, baking soda, baking powder, sea salt, cinnamon, and nutmeg. Add the wet ingredients to the dry and mix together, but don't overmix. Transfer to a 9 x 5 x 3-inch loaf pan that has been lightly sprayed with nonstick spray.

Bake for 1 hour (depending on your oven, it could take 10 minutes extra to feel springy on the top).

Remove from the oven and let the banana bread cool for 10 minutes. Carefully invert and remove the bread. Let it cool completely before slicing.

Per serving (¹/₁₂ of recipe): 166 calories, 3 g protein, 39 g carbohydrate, 20 g sugar, 1 g fat, 3% calories from fat, 2 g fiber, 226 mg sodium

Recipe by Christine Waltermyer

Oatmeal Raisin Cookies

MAKES 18 COOKIES

½ cup unbleached white flour

½ cup whole wheat or spelt flour

1 cup quick-cooking oats

½ teaspoon baking powder

½ teaspoon cinnamon

Pinch of nutmeg

¼ teaspoon sea salt

¾ cup mashed bananas (about 2 bananas)

⅓ cup maple syrup

1 teaspoon vanilla extract

⅓ cup raisins

Preheat the oven to 350°F. In a large bowl, whisk together the flours, oats, baking powder, cinnamon, nutmeg, and sea salt. In a small bowl, combine the bananas, maple syrup, and vanilla.

Add the wet ingredients to the dry ingredients. Mix well, but don't overmix. Stir in the raisins.

Place tablespoon-size cookies on a baking sheet lined with parchment paper. Using wet hands, press the cookies flat into nice cookie shapes. Bake for 12 minutes.

Per cookie (¹⁄₁₈ of recipe): 74 calories, 2 g protein, 16 g carbohydrate, 6 g sugar, 0.5 g fat, 5% calories from fat, 1 g fiber, 48 mg sodium

Recipe by Christine Waltermyer

References

1. Barnard ND, Levin SM, Yokoyama Y. A systematic review and meta-analysis of changes in body weight in clinical trials of vegetarian diets. *J Acad Nutr Diet*. 2015;115:954–969.

2. Barnard ND, Scialli AR, Turner-McGrievy G, Lanou AJ, Glass J. The effects of a low-fat, plant-based dietary intervention on body weight, metabolism, and insulin sensitivity. *Am J Med*. 2005;118:991–997.

3. Jenkins DJ, Kendall CW, Marchie A, et al. Direct comparison of a dietary portfolio of cholesterol-lowering foods with a statin in hypercholesterolemic participants. *Am J Clin Nutr*. 2005;81:380–387.

4. Barnard ND, Cohen J, Jenkins DJ, et al. A low-fat vegan diet and a conventional diabetes diet in the treatment of type 2 diabetes: a randomized, controlled, 74-week clinical trial. *Am J Clin Nutr*. 2009;89(suppl):1588S–1596S.

5. Yokoyama Y, Nishimura K, Barnard ND, et al. Vegetarian diets and blood pressure: a meta-analysis. *JAMA Intern Med*. 2014;174:577–587.

6. Lu W, Chen H, Niu Y, Wu H, Xia D, Wu Y. Dairy products intake and cancer mortality risk: a meta-analysis of 11 population-based cohort studies. *Nutr J*. 2016;15:91–102.

7. Chlebowski RT, Blackburn GL, Thomson CA, et al. Dietary fat reduction and breast cancer outcome: interim efficacy results from the Women's Intervention Nutrition Study. *J Natl Cancer Inst.* 2006;98:1767–1776.

8. Pierce JP, Stefanick ML, Flatt SW, et al. Greater survival after breast cancer in physically active women with high vegetable–fruit intake regardless of obesity. *J Clin Oncol.* 2007;25:2345–2351.

9. Ornish D, Weidner G, Fair WR, et al. Intensive lifestyle changes may affect the progression of prostate cancer. *J Urol.* 2005;174:1065–1070.

10. Wu AH, Yu MC, Tseng CC, Pike MC. Epidemiology of soy exposures and breast cancer risk. *Br J Cancer.* 2008;98:9–14.

11. Chen M, Rao Y, Zheng Y, et al. Association between soy isoflavone intake and breast cancer risk for pre- and post-menopausal women: a meta-analysis of epidemiological studies. *PLoS ONE.* 2014;9(2):e89288.

12. Nechuta SJ, Caan BJ, Chen WY, et al. Soy food intake after diagnosis of breast cancer and survival: an in-depth analysis of combined evidence from cohort studies of US and Chinese women. *Am J Clin Nutr.* 2012;96:123–132.

13. Morris MC, Evans DA, Bienias JL, et al. Dietary fats and the risk of incident Alzheimer disease. *Arch Neurol.* 2003;60:194–200.

14. Erickson KI, Voss MW, Prakash RS, et al. Exercise training increases size of hippocampus and improves memory. *Proc Natl Acad Sci U S A.* 2011;108:3017–3022.

15. Turner-McGrievy GM, Barnard ND, Cohen J, Jenkins DJ, Gloede L, Green AA. Changes in nutrient intake and dietary quality among participants with type 2 diabetes following a low-fat vegan diet or a conventional diabetes diet for 22 weeks. *J Am Diet Assoc.* 2008;108:1636–1645.

16. Melina V, Craig W, Levin S. Position of the Academy of Nutrition and Dietetics: vegetarian diets. *J Acad Nutr Diet.* 2016;116:1970–1980.

17. Carter JP, Furman T, Hutcheson HR. Preeclampsia and reproductive performance in a community of vegans. *South Med J.* 1987;80:692–697.

18. Wolfram T. Healthy Weight during Pregnancy. Eat Right, Academy of Nutrition and Dietetics. http://www.eatright.org/health/pregnancy/prenatal-wellness/healthy-weight-during-pregnancy. Accessed November 22, 2017.

19. McCloskey K, Ponsonby AL, Collier F, et al. The association between higher maternal pre-pregnancy body mass index and increased birth weight, adiposity and inflammation in the newborn. *Pediatr Obes.* 2016 Oct 9. doi:10.1111/ijpo.12187. [Epub ahead of print]

20. Clyne PS, Kulczycki A Jr. Human breast milk contains bovine IgG: relationship to infant colic? *Pediatrics.* 1991;87:439–444.

21. Te Morenga L, Montez JM. Health effects of saturated and trans-fatty acid intake in children and adolescents: systematic review and meta-analysis. *PLoS One.* 2017;12:e0186672.

22. Christakis NA, Fowler JH. The spread of obesity in a large social network over 32 years. *N Engl J Med.* 2007;357:370–379.

Index

About the Author

Neal D. Barnard, MD, FACC, is perhaps the world's most respected authority on vegan diets. He is a faculty member of the George Washington University School of Medicine and president of the Physicians Committee for Responsible Medicine. Dr. Barnard's research, funded by the US government, revolutionized the dietary approach to type 2 diabetes, and his findings have influenced the policies of the US Dietary Guidelines Advisory Committee, the American Diabetes Association, and the American Medical Association. In 2015, he was named a fellow of the American College of Cardiology, and in 2016, he received the American College of Lifestyle Medicine's Trailblazer Award. Dr. Barnard is editor-in-chief of the *Nutrition Guide for Clinicians*, a nutrition textbook given to all medical students in the United States.